Were You There?

03/06/2026
To Enn w/ lots of good wishes & fond memories of our work together to uncover & tell stories long forgotten!

Were You There?

A Biography of Emma Wakefield-Paillet

by Phebe Hayes and Margaret Simon

2025
University of Louisiana at Lafayette Press

© 2024 by Phebe Hayes and Margaret Simon
All rights reserved
ISBN 13 (paper): 978-1-959569-19-0

http://ulpress.org
University of Louisiana at Lafayette Press
P.O. Box 43558
Lafayette, LA 70504-3558

Library of Congress Cataloging-in-Publication Data

Names: Hayes, Phebe, 1954- author. | Simon, Margaret Gibson, author.
Title: Were you there? : A biography of Emma Wakefield-Paillet / by Phebe Hayes and Margaret Simon.
Description: Lafayette, LA : University of Louisiana at Lafayette Press, 2025. | Audience: Ages 13 and up | Audience: Grades 7-9
Identifiers: LCCN 2024054334 | ISBN 9781959569190 (paperback)
Subjects: LCSH: Wakefield-Paillet, Emma, 1868-1946. | African American women physicians--Louisiana--New Orleans--Biography--Juvenile literature. | African American women physicians--California--San Francisco--Biography--Juvenile literature. | African American women--Louisiana--New Iberia--Biography--Juvenile literature. | African American women physicians--Poetry. | LCGFT: Biographies. | Poetry.
Classification: LCC R154.W35 H39 2025 | DDC 610.92 [B]--dc23/eng/20250213
LC record available at https://lccn.loc.gov/2024054334

Cover art by Clifford Etienne

*To New Orleans genealogist Jari Honora, for leading me
to the remarkable Dr. Emma Wakefield-Paillet.*

—Phebe

*To women pioneers whose stories we tell
and those whose stories we have yet to discover.*

—Margaret

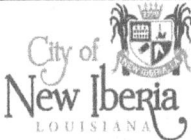

City of New Iberia, LOUISIANA

Mayoral Proclamation

WHEREAS, Dr. Emma Wakefield-Paillet was born in the City of New Iberia, Louisiana on November 21, 1868 to state Senator Samuel and Mrs. Amelia Valentine Wakefield both natives of New Iberia; and

WHEREAS, She went on to study medicine at the Medical Department of New Orleans University where she graduated with honors in 1897; and

WHEREAS, She was the sole female of sixty-eight applicants (including four Blacks) who sat for licensure with the Louisiana State Board of Medical Examiners in 1897; and

WHEREAS, Special mention was made of her exceptional performance on the examination in the LSBME Board Minutes; and

WHEREAS, She is the first African American female to practice medicine in the State of Louisiana, having been awarded a medical license by the Louisiana Board of Medical Examiners on April 15, 1897; and

WHEREAS, She is the first African American female to practice medicine in New Orleans, Louisiana having opened a medical practice at 1233 North Villere and Esplanade in 1898; and

WHEREAS, An official state historical marker commemorating the trailblazing accomplishments of Dr. Emma Wakefield-Paillet will be placed in her hometown of New Iberia, Louisiana on November 3, 2018;

NOW THEREFORE, I, Mayor Freddie DeCourt, by virtue of the authority vested in me by the laws of the City of New Iberia, do hereby proclaim November 3, 2018 as

DR. EMMA WAKEFIELD-PAILLET DAY
In New Iberia, Louisiana.

IN WITNESS WHEREOF, I hereunto have set my hand and caused the seal of the City of New Iberia be affixed this 3rd of November, 2018

Freddie DeCourt, Mayor
City of New Iberia, Louisiana

Table of Contents

Preface xiii
    Were You There? xvii

The Birth of Emma Wakefield 1
    Birth of Courage 3

An Industrious Father 5
    Under Swaying Sugarcane 7
    Frederick Speaks of Freedom 9
    Train to the Senate 11
    We, the People 13

The Importance of Education 15
    Wakefield Institute Destroyed by Tornado 19

A Family Familiar with Death 21
    Samuel Wakefield's "Suicide," 1883 25
    Aurora Hail, and All the Thousand Dies 27

Malaria Claims Sister Amelia 29
    With tears and toiling breath, for Amelia 31

Another Tragedy Strikes 33
    Ballad for Sammie 35
    They Come for Adolph 36

The Wakefields Leave New Iberia 37

Embracing Education 39
    Making a Choice 41

Emma Becomes a Physician 43
    Phillis Wheatley Club 47
    Riding Home on the Streetcar 51

"Exceptionally Excellent" Emma 53
    Graduation Sestina 55
    Some People Say 57

The Wakefields Leave Louisiana 59
   Riding the Train in the Dark 61
   Ode to the Steam Locomotive: 1900 62
   Wedding Eintou 63

"Passing for White" 65
   San Francisco, 1901 67

Another Sister Lost 69
   Invictus 71

Cholera Claims Adolph Wakefield 73
   Thirteen Ways of Looking at Cholera 77

Returning to Louisiana 81
   Sonnet After the San Francisco Earthquake, 1906 83
   Today I Will Praise 84

The End of Emma's Life 87
   I Know Who I Am 89

Timeline 92

Historical Background 95

Poetic Forms and Inspiration 105

Educational Guide 109

Critical Thinking Questions by Section 111

Pre-Reading and Post-Reading Word Sort 117

Timeline Activity 119

Write a Poem 121

Acknowledgments 123

About the Authors 125

A Note to Readers

The time period in which Emma Wakefield-Paillet lived, the late 1800s and early 1900s, was often turbulent and dangerous. This was especially true for people of color. As such, this work deals with difficult subject matter, including racial violence, discrimination, and suicide. It may be unsuitable for some readers.

PREFACE

This collaboration recalls the life of one of New Iberia, Louisiana's hidden historical figures through prose and poetry. While prose can tell a story, poetry can stir an emotion. Some of the poems are new works based on historical information. Other poems may echo a past work using words, phrases, and forms inspired by poems, songs, or speeches of the time. We hope that this book helps you learn about an unsung heroine as well as touches your heart and leads you to respond with your own poems. Moreover, we hope that you will understand and appreciate a little of the process historians use to uncover hidden stories.

From the beginning, our aim has been to tell the inspiring story of Dr. Emma Wakefield-Paillet, the first woman of any ethnicity to earn a medical degree from a Louisiana medical school (1897).[1] In addition, she was the first African American woman to be licensed to practice medicine in Louisiana and the first African American woman to establish her own medical practice in New Orleans.

As the researcher on this project, Phebe Hayes first became aware of Dr. Wakefield-Paillet through the work of New Orleans historian and genealogist Jari Honora. We are grateful to him and the other founders and staff of CreoleGen, the online blog of the Creole Genealogical and Historical Association, for bringing this New Iberia native to the public's attention. Researching Dr. Wakefield-Paillet further, Phebe learned just how important she was in a time and profession dominated by men, and mainly White men at that. After graduating with honors in 1897 from the Medical Department of New Orleans University, she sat for the licensure exam administered by the Louisiana State Board of Medical Examiners. The only female in a field of sixty-eight candidates, Dr. Wakefield-Paillet distinguished herself so well on the

---

1. The first woman to practice medicine in Louisiana was Dr. Elizabeth Magnus Cohen, who was born in New York City and studied medicine at the Female Medical College of Pennsylvania. Dr. Cohen began practicing medicine in New Orleans in 1857, forty years before Dr. Wakefield-Paillet earned her medical degree.

test that her performance was singled out for special mention in the board's meeting minutes.

Incredibly, despite being a native and lifelong resident of Iberia Parish, Phebe had never heard of Dr. Wakefield-Paillet or her amazing family until she came across the CreoleGen blog post. Intrigued by the story of this New Iberia physician previously unknown to her, Phebe sought more information about Dr. Wakefield-Paillet and her family. Her research brought her to online sites like www.newspapers.com and www.ancestry.com, in addition to the resources at CreoleGen. She visited or consulted with staff at archives, museums, libraries, and courthouses, including the Tulane University Amistad Center, the Dillard University archives, the Historic New Orleans Collection, the Young-Sanders Center for the Study of the War Between the States in Louisiana, and the Clerks of Court of Iberia and St. Martin Parishes. Phebe also contacted the state medical boards in Louisiana and California to verify Dr. Wakefield-Paillet's medical practices in each state. She examined publications and online posts of the National Medical Association and the American Medical Association, as well as books (some out of print) regarding the history of Straight University and New Orleans University. She attended meetings and conferences of state genealogy and historical organizations such as the Louisiana Creole Research Association annual conferences and the Imperial St. Landry Genealogy Society of Opelousas, Louisiana, for information about the Wakefield and Paillet families.

To understand the historical context of the times Dr. Wakefield-Paillet and her family lived, Phebe revisited the periods of Reconstruction and Jim Crow segregation. She conducted telephone interviews with renowned historians and Reconstruction-era scholars such as Dr. Eric Foner of Columbia University and Dr. Charles Vincent of Southern University and A&M College. She reached out to relatives of Dr. Wakefield-Paillet's husband, Joseph Oscar Paillet, who provided stories and pictures of the couple taken in 1926 San Francisco. Finally, she contacted a descendant of Louis Charles Roudanez, who was founder and publisher of the country's first African American newspaper, *L'Union*

(1862–1864), and the first African American daily newspaper, the *New Orleans Tribune* (1864–1869), for any information he might have in his family archive about the Wakefields.

Phebe's research yielded evidence of Dr. Wakefield-Paillet's education, including her graduation from Straight University with honors and her admission to the Medical Department at New Orleans University with two other young women. Both dropped out of the program before completing their medical degrees. Details of her 1897 medical school graduation ceremony, such as the names of her classmates and professors, were also uncovered. Her research also yielded concrete evidence of Dr. Wakefield-Paillet as the first woman to graduate from a Louisiana medical school and the first African American woman to be licensed to practice medicine in Louisiana. Phebe also found an ad Dr. Wakefield-Paillet placed announcing the relocation of her medical practice to 1233 North Villere St. in the 1898 New Orleans *Times-Democrat*. So far, Phebe has been unable to conclusively identify the location of Dr. Wakefield-Paillet's first office. It is probable that she initially saw patients at her 1020 Orleans Avenue home, where she lived at the time of her medical school graduation.

Dr. Wakefield-Paillet's story is compelling. Born only three years after the end of slavery in southern Louisiana and one month after the creation of her home parish, Iberia Parish, her story spans both the Reconstruction and Jim Crow eras of United States history. We include those difficult historical periods in the telling of her story. Because members of Dr. Wakefield-Paillet's family figure prominently in those periods of history, their stories are also included in this book.

It is important to note that while Margaret Simon used Black authors as inspiration for Emma's voice in poems, these poems are not historical documents from the time. They are verses to convey the emotions Emma may have been experiencing during the events of her life.

In 2017, Phebe founded the Iberia African American Historical Society (IAAHS). Its purpose is to research, teach, and commemorate the history of African Americans in the parish. To honor Dr. Wakefield-Paillet's legacy, the historical society installed a state marker in New Iberia's historic district on November 18, 2018. That marker is located on Main Street, adjacent to the city's town square, Bouligny Plaza. Between that marker and this book, it is our hope that Dr. Wakefield-Paillet's legacy will be remembered and honored forever.

> Phebe A. Hayes, PhD
> Founder & President
> The Iberia African American Historical Society
>
> Margaret Simon, MEd, NBCT
> Teacher
> The Iberia Parish Public School System

Were You There?

Were you there
when Momma held my hand?
when she walked with me to school?
when she knelt down in the sand?
when neighbors could be so cruel?

Were you there
when infants were enslaved at birth?
when my people cut the cane?
when shadows veiled the earth?
when teardrops fell like rain?

Were you there
when we finally broke the chains?
when our hollow cries were heard?
when mothers' sons were slain?
when I could read the Word?

Oh, Lord, were you there?

Inspired by "Were You There (When They Crucified My Lord)," an African American spiritual, or religious song. The first known printing of the song dates back to 1899, though it was likely sung for decades before that.

November 21, 1868

THE BIRTH OF EMMA WAKEFIELD

The fall of 1868 was an exciting time in the lives of Samuel and Amelia Wakefield. The couple eagerly awaited the birth of their fourth child and the first to be born into freedom. The Civil War had finally ended in 1865, after four long, horrible years of violence. President Lincoln's Emancipation Proclamation had declared that enslaved people in the South would now be free, with the exception of those living in areas of Federal occupation. New Iberia was one of these areas. Shortly after, Congress had passed the Thirteenth Amendment, which formally made slavery illegal, except as punishment for a crime. And just a few months before Emma's birth, in July 1868, the Fourteenth Amendment proclaimed that all people born in the United States are citizens of the country.

Emma's birth represented a new era for the Wakefields. Unlike the rest of the family, this new infant would be born with all the rights and privileges of native-born citizens. She would never experience the pains, limitations, and indignities of enslavement. Samuel and Amelia would see to it that their new child, like their other children, would be well-educated and prepared for the opportunities of post-emancipation America.

Meanwhile, progress was happening all around them. Voters elected African American men to important political and governmental positions. Freedmen established businesses, purchased property, and provided educational opportunities for their children. In fact, the state government called for the creation of a new parish around the same time as the birth of the new baby, and the Wakefields' hometown, New Iberia, was slated to become the parish seat. On October 30, 1868, a legislative act officially established Iberia Parish. Emma was born one month later, on November 21, 1868. Three additional children joined the family later: Samuel Jr. (Sammie) in 1872 and twins Mary Adele and Mary Victoria in 1876.

BIRTH OF COURAGE

As the hot summer air
cools into fall,
while Samuel Wakefield hammers
another wooden barrel for his weekly count,

>I am born, fourth child, third girl,
>the color of copper and ash.

Amelia and Samuel hear my cry of courage,
>determination wrapped in a swaddling blanket.

On November 21, 1868, I am as newborn as
Iberia Parish, Louisiana,
birthed from the muddy Bayou Teche,
emerging into emancipation,
proof that the bayou sculpts
a strong will.

Fourteenth Senatorial District Convention.

Delegates to this convention met at Plaquemine on Saturday, August 15, the following parishes being represented as follows:

Iberville—Basile Craig, George Randolph, Alcee Johnson, Gabriel Bess, Marcelin Napoleon, Charles Dedrick, Dr. King Holt, James L. Cole. Alternates: William Whittaker, John H. Jackson, Louis Johnson, July Coakly, Alfred Butler, Isaac Martin, Z. C. Brooks, Aaron Parker.

West Baton Rouge—Rufus B. Caldwell, Stephen Colwell, Hon. T. T. Allain. Alternates: Frank Delaney, Oscar Holt, William A. Colwell.

St. Martin—Charles Neuven, Jefferson Vavasseur, Ernest Delahoussaye, Hon. Victor Rochon.

Iberia—L. A. Snaer, Samuel Wakefield, E. H. Riddell.

The votes for the parish of Iberia were cast by L. A. Snaer, the other delegates being absent.

At the request of the delegates Hon. T. T. Allain, of West Baton Rouge, called the convention to order.

This article in the *New Orleans Republican* from Tuesday, August 18, 1874 describes the convention that voted to create Iberia Parish. New Iberia, the Iberia Parish seat, is where Emma would spend her childhood. Samuel Wakefield is listed as one of the delegates from Iberia Parish.

1874–1876

AN INDUSTRIOUS FATHER

Emma's father, Samuel, made a decent living at various times as a cooper (or barrel maker), grocer, and newspaper co-owner. To achieve the goals he and his wife, Amelia, had for their family, he chose to pursue new opportunities after emancipation. Samuel aligned himself with the Republican Party of the time and sought and won several political offices, including tax collector, a seat on the New Iberia Mayor's Board of Trustees, and the Louisiana state senate. He was also appointed as a trustee of Straight University and as one of two required Black commissioners on the Iberia Parish Public School Board. Samuel also received a presidential appointment as postmaster of Iberia Parish. He was the first African American to serve in that position. Eventually, he was appointed as a deputy naval officer in New Orleans. In this position, he was responsible for inspecting ships as they came into the port of New Orleans and traveled up and down the Mississippi River. He also collected duties, or taxes, on the goods these ships brought in from other regions. Naval officers were considered very respectable, and Samuel must have had a strong reputation in order to be chosen for the position.

Throughout Emma's childhood, she and her siblings benefited greatly as the offspring of such an industrious father.

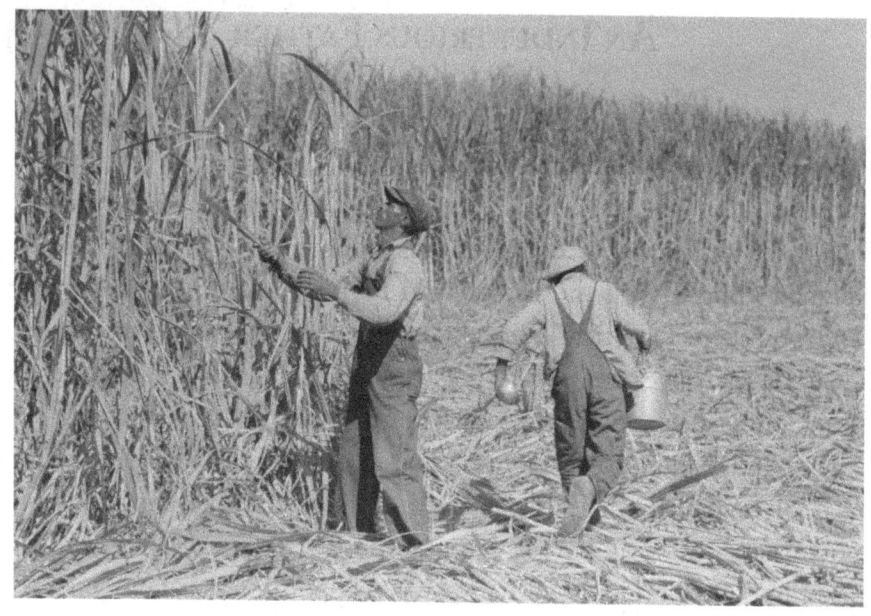

Many of the farms around New Iberia grew sugarcane, like the one shown in this image taken in 1938. Often, formerly enslaved people performed the difficult labor of harvesting the sugarcane.

Source: *Sugarcane cutter and waterboy in field near New Iberia, Louisiana* (1938) by Russell Lee. Courtesy of the Library of Congress, Prints & Photographs Division, Farm Security Administration/Office of War Information Black-and-White Negatives.

Under Swaying Sugarcane

Under swaying sugarcane,
Daddy envisions a better life.
After emancipation, opportunities
rise like smoke from the mills
spreading sweetness
to his tongue.
Every day he climbs another rung of the ladder,
a postmaster, then a tax collector,
from colored school district director
to state senator. Each new position
a step toward better.
My father tastes success.
He aspires
to make a difference in Iberia Parish,
a wave of equal access
to jobs, education, a future
for his children, for me.
Little does he know his days are numbered.
Little does he know a rumble
of hatred and disgrace spreads
beneath the cane.
Little does he know ...

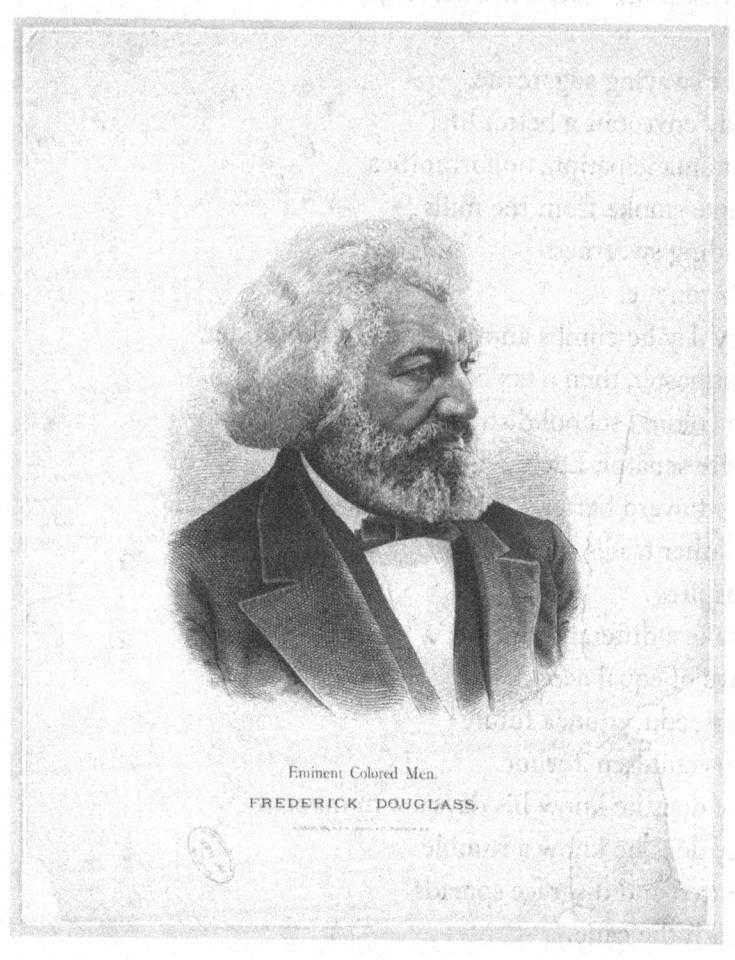

Frederick Douglass was a respected leader during the Reconstruction Era, and his speeches inspired many people, like Emma's father.

Source: *Eminent Colored Men. Frederick Douglass / F.F.; Moss Eng. Co. N.Y.* Moss Engraving Company and John Wesley Cromwell (1884).
Courtesy of the Library of Congress.

Frederick Speaks of Freedom

Daddy reads beside me
a new speech from Frederick Douglass.

Words of hope and freedom
whisper to me
from Daddy's chair.
Mr. Douglass says
If a Black man is free,
freed by the law,
If your heart be as my heart,
liberty has been given.

Daddy looks up from the paper.
Mr. Douglass writes wisdom. His words are strong, inspire
a desire in me to get involved in government.

He speaks to crowds of people
of freedom and rights
of Blacks for liberty.

His words move me, like Daddy,
make me wriggle in my skin
and dream of a road
to Frederick's freedom.

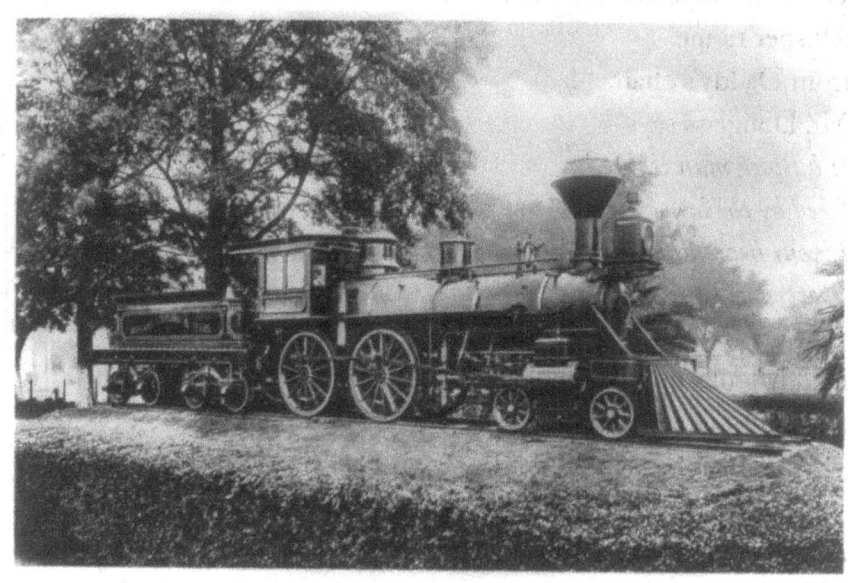

In his new role as a state senator, Emma's father had to travel from New Iberia to New Orleans, the state capital at the time. He might have taken a train like this to get there.

Source: Locomotive Sabine, part of Charles Morgan's Louisiana & Texas Railroad line. Courtesy of the Library of Congress.

Train to the Senate

Momma holds my hand
while we walk with Daddy to the train station.
He's wearing his best suit
heading to New Orleans
for his first session of the state senate.

Daddy's face never glowed so proud.
From the window of the train
he looks my way,
promising

to stand   as a free man
to carry   the legacy of President Lincoln
to confront   prejudice
to make   history.

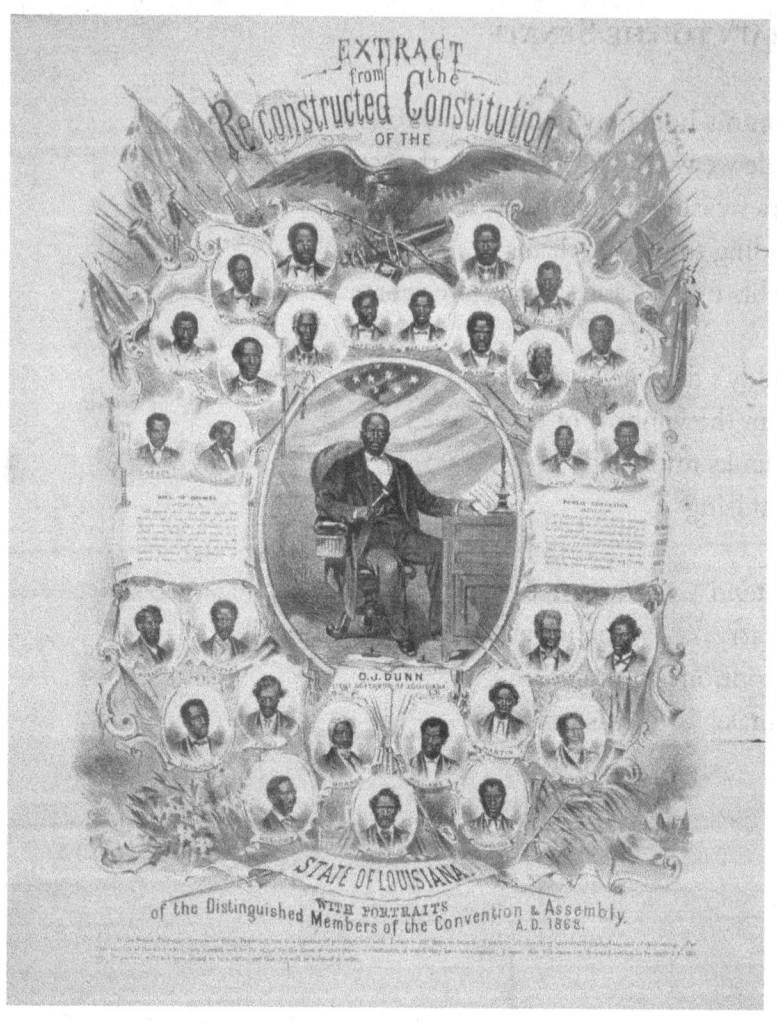

During Reconstruction, African American men were finally able to hold political positions in Louisiana. Many were elected to the state legislature, and one, Oscar J. Dunn, served as the state's first African American lieutenant governor. This print from 1868 shows the portraits of those distinguished African American members of the constitutional convention, who worked to create the new state constitution in 1868.

Source: *Extract from the reconstructed Constitution of the state of Louisiana, with portraits of the distinguished members of the Convention & Assembly, A.D. Louisiana, 1868.* Courtesy of the Library of Congress.

WE, THE PEOPLE
after Rita Williams-Garcia

We, the people
lift our voices,
carry them forth,
speak of freedom.

We, the people
appreciate our minds,
march toward the dream,
invite others in.

We, the people
reject ignorance,
question prejudice,
protect our rights.

Daddy, are we the people?

Yes, my child
All of us.
Not some of us.
We are the people,
you and I,
your brothers,
your sisters,
your teacher,
our preacher,
and all the singing voices of the choir.

We are the people!

Inspiration for this poem came from Rita Williams Garcia's essay "We, the People" in *We Rise, We Resist, We Raise our Voices*, edited by Wade Hudson and Cheryl Willis Hudson, 2018.

1874

The Importance of Education

More than anything, Samuel and Amelia Wakefield wanted their seven children, including Emma, to be educated and prepared to assume leadership roles in post-Civil War Louisiana. The period of rebuilding after the Civil War became known as Reconstruction. During this time, legislatures across the South began instituting policies that granted African Americans more rights. The Freedmen's Bureau, created by Congress, worked to provide food, clothing, and other basic needs for formerly enslaved people, as well as to help them find new jobs and places to live.

Thanks to these efforts, for the first time, African Americans could legally access education. Aid came from northern organizations and philanthropists who sent funds and teachers (White and Black) to build and staff schools in the South. Reconstruction-era schools in Iberia Parish were all segregated, meaning separated by race. Despite the 1868 Louisiana state constitution that provided for integrated public schools (open to all races), segregation remained a reality in New Iberia. It is unlikely that Emma and her siblings ever attended school with White children. Schools in Louisiana remained segregated until 1968.

Samuel worked tirelessly to provide the children of Iberia's freedmen access to a quality education. In the 1860s, he was appointed as one of the Black commissioners of the Iberia Parish public schools. Early in the creation of public education in Iberia, he and his wife allowed the parish public school board to use part of their home as a school for Black girls. By 1874, he had built his own private preparatory school, Wakefield Institute, located on Bank Street near his home. In a printed flier, he announced the imminent opening of the new school and recruited faculty and students. Sadly, a tornado blew through town in 1874 and destroyed the new two-story building. There is no evidence that the school ever opened. That same year, Samuel was appointed to the Board of Trustees of Straight University in New Orleans. Classes at Straight University ranged from elementary to college level. As a trustee, Emma's father recruited children from Iberia Parish to attend the preparatory school. All the Wakefield children eventually attended Straight University.

Samuel made extra payment to Straight University to provide his children with music education. All Emma's siblings, except young Sammie, played musical instruments. Emma took piano lessons and eventually became an excellent pianist.

WAKEFIELD UNIVERSITY.

This University is located in New Iberia, La., on Bank Avenue; comprising Normal, Collegiate, Theological and Needle Work Departments; vested in a body of Trustees, representing different religious denominations. Its desire is the education of young men and women, without regard to race, color or previous condition; and as education is the best fitness for citizenship, and many Teachers are wanted, therefore we appeal in the name of religion and humanity to all lovers of piety to aid us in this important work. Clergymen, Teachers and District Superintendents throughout the parishes can do much good in directing the attention of students to this institution, and by putting them in correspondence with the Secretary.

BOARD OF TRUSTEES.

SAMUEL WAKEFIELD, *President.*
ARISTIDE NORMAN, *Vice President.*
JOHN PICKET, Jr.,
THOMAS HALCOM,
BENJAMIN KEENAN,
OLIVIER BOUTTE,
PETER LODGE,
SAMUEL KELLER,
Rev. S. W. ROGERS, *Secretary.*
JOHN PICKET, *Treasurer.*
Rev. DAVID JOHNSON,
PAUL MARTIN,
BENJAMIN KELLER.

UNIVERSITE WAKEFIELD.

Cette Université est située à la Nouvelle-Ibérie, sur l'Avenue Bank; comprenant les branches Normal, Theologique, Classique et Travail d'Aiguille, sous la direction d'un corps représentant des différentes sectes réligieuses. L'objet est l'éducation des jeunes gens, de toutes races et conditions; et comme l'éducation est une des qualités principales pour être bon citoyen, et que nous souffrons beaucoup de la necessité des Tuteurs dignes de confiance; nous appelons au nom de la réligion et l'humanité, à tous les honnêtes gens de nous assister dans ce travail important. Les ministres, professeurs et Superintendents de District sont priés d'appeler l'attention des étudiants à cette institution, et les mettrent en rapport avec le Secrétaire.

DIRECTEURS.

SAMUEL WAKEFIELD, *Président.*
ARISTIDE NORMAN, *Vice Président.*
JOHN PICKET, Jr.,
THOMAS HALCOM,
BENJAMIN KEENAN.
OLIVIER BOUTTE,
PETER LODGE,
SAMUEL KELLER,
Rev. S. W. ROGERS, *Secrétaire.*
JOHN PICKET, *Tresorier.*
Rev. DAVID JOHNSON,
PAUL MARTIN,
BENJAMIN KELLER.

Printed at the "TIMES" Office, New Iberia, La.

Samuel Wakefield had fliers printed and distributed around New Iberia advertising for his new school. Note that the flier was printed in English as well as French, because many people in the area spoke French as their first language.

Source: Amistad Research Center

WAKEFIELD INSTITUTE DESTROYED BY TORNADO

Daddy's dream
blew away during the night.

He cries   *My beloved institute is gone,*
              dead in the path of a tornado.

Thunder of his voice
wakes me. My footsteps rotate
around his anger.
Words swirl through the air.

        How will I educate my children now?

Daddy thinks of Reverend Adams,
his school in New Orleans.

        A free, safe place to learn,
        where all children are treated fairly,
        no matter their color.
        Adolph will go.

My older brother takes the Morgan Train
to Straight University. He'll study
and learn and take music lessons.

Daddy, can I go with Dolph?
        All in good time, my dear,
        all in good time.

1883

A Family Familiar with Death

By the time Emma was fifteen years old, she was used to her father's long absences as he traveled to and from New Orleans. Yet one day, he did not come home as expected. Soon, the family received horrible news: Emma's father had been found dead. The news that their beloved father was gone came as a shock to the whole family.

Even more disturbing, newspapers began to print stories claiming he had died by suicide. The family could not believe it. They read and reread the articles but knew their father would never do such a thing.

Emma was devastated. She refused to believe that her dear father had killed himself. Her father had many friends, but he also had many enemies. Was it possible that his suicide was staged? The only eyewitness was her father's brother-in-law, Henderson Ford, who was married to his sister, Mary Alice. Could he have been bullied into saying that it was a suicide? According to the initial coroner's report, he had shot himself twice in the head. How could that be possible? The first bullet to the head would have left her father unconscious, even if it hadn't killed him. Emma relied heavily on her oldest brother, Adolph (called A. J. by his family and friends), other family members, and friends to get through the trauma of her father's death.

Emma's mother also needed to be strong. Samuel's death made her a widow with seven children to care for. Through her tears, Emma witnessed her mother's might and resilience. Sadly, in the coming years, Emma would again see her mother's tears, after the early deaths of two of the Wakefield children.

Still, Emma saw that despite such devastating tragedies, her mother kept her family together and saw to it that her children completed their education.

LOCAL INTELLIGENCE.

THE REGULAR RECORD OF CURRENT EVENTS THROUGHOUT THE CITY.

SUICIDAL SUCCESS.

Ex-State Senator Samuel Wakefield Blows His Brains Out.

Samuel Wakefield, the colored ex-State Senator from Iberia parish, suicided yesterday morning at 8 o'clock, at the residence of Henderson Ford, his brother-in-law, No. 329 Howard street. Wakefield arrived on Wednesday night from New Iberia, and was accommodated with a room at Ford's house. During the night he appeared despondent and morose, and early in the morning arose and dressed himself. At 8 o'clock he walked out into the yard and a few seconds afterward the report of a pistol was heard. Ford rushed out and found Wakefield lying behind the cistern. As he approached him Wakefield raised himself on his elbow and placing the muzzle of his revolver to his right temple, pulled the trigger, killing himself instantly.

Deputy Coroner Dr. Archinard, viewed the body, and found that the first shot had grazed the scalp, while the second entered the brain. He gave a certificate of suicide, and the remains were taken charge of by the family and will be sent to New Iberia.

Wakefield was a man of some prominence. He was born in St. Martin, but established himself as a political leader in Iberia parish. He was appointed tax collector by the Republicans, and in 1876 was elected to the State Senate and sat in the Packard Legislature. Upon the organization under Gov. Nicholls he was deposed, and his seat given to Mr. Wailes. He was then appointed deputy naval officer under Dumont and served until December 4, 1882, when he was removed. Since then he had been laboring to obtain employment, but being unsuccessful, gave up hope and ended his life by his own hand. On his person a letter from Washington was found, setting forth that the writer had interviewed Senator Kellogg in his behalf and that the Senator had promised to use his influence with Gen. Badger.

Wakefield had been in ill health for some time, and his friends state that his sickness, together with his financial embarrassment, caused him to commit the rash act. The deceased leaves a wife and seven children.

Source: *The Times-Democrat*, New Orleans, Louisiana, February 2, 1883

SUICIDAL SUCCESS

Samuel Wakefield, the colored ex-State Senator from Iberia Parish, suicided yesterday morning at 8 o'clock, at the residence of Henderson Ford, his brother-in-law, No. 329 Howard Street. Wakefield arrived on Wednesday night from New Iberia and was accommodated with a room at Ford's house. During the night he appeared despondent and morose, and early in the morning arose and dressed himself. At 8 o'clock he walked out into the yard and a few seconds afterward the report of a pistol was heard. Ford rushed out and found Wakefield lying behind the cistern. As he approached him, Wakefield raised himself on his elbow and placing the muzzle of his revolver to his right temple, pulled the trigger, killing himself instantly.

Deputy Coroner Dr. Archinard viewed the body and found that the first shot had grazed the scalp, while the second entered the brain. He gave a certificate of suicide, and the remains were taken charge of by the family and will be sent to New Iberia.

Samuel Wakefield's "Suicide," 1883

Stop!
Stop all the noise.
I bury my face into my pillow and scream.
Stop saying

my daddy is dead.
My daddy *shot himself in the head?*
No, not my daddy.

My daddy was righteous
and true
and full of grit.

He'd say,
Emma, dear,
you were made to break free.
To be more than me.

Mama holds my face in her hands,
wipes vinegar tears that stain my cheeks,
and looks hard into my eyes.

We will carry on, child.
We must carry on.

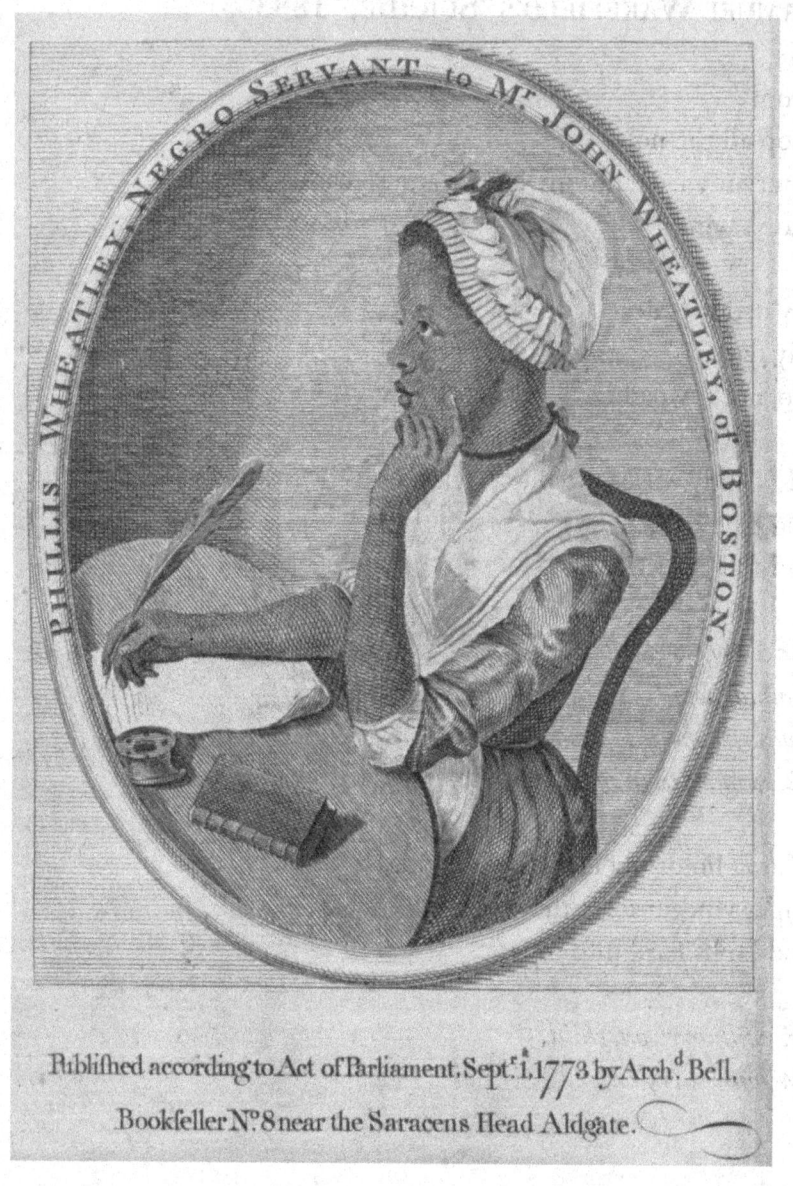

Phillis Wheatley, the first African American to publish a book of poetry.

Source: Library of Congress

Aurora Hail, and All the Thousand Dies

> Over my sweet mother, **Aurora**
> rains tears as we **hail**
> his passing casket **and**
> **all**
> our lives change. Among **the**
> **thousand**
> buried here, Daddy is my own who **dies.**

The line for this golden shovel poem, "Aurora hail, and all the thousand dies," is from "An Hymn to the Morning" by Phillis Wheatley, published in 1773. Phillis Wheatley was the first African American, and one of the first women in colonial America, to have a book of poetry published. She was born in West Africa and sold into slavery as a young girl. Soon after her book was published, she was freed by her enslavers. President George Washington was among those who praised her poetry.

1887

MALARIA CLAIMS SISTER AMELIA

Over the next few years, the Wakefields resumed their regular activities, despite their grief. In the spring and summer months, they looked forward to spending time outdoors. Sometimes Emma and her siblings took wagon excursions out to Avery Island for a day of picnicking, crabbing, and fishing. They particularly enjoyed activities held each year at the family church, St. Paul Congregational Church located on Madison Street. (This was later renamed Pershing Street.) Her father had cofounded St. Paul and had been one of its most influential members.

Yet, these outdoor days always came with a risk of mosquitos. Growing up, Emma could not stand these buzzing, annoying pests. Their bites itched and left raised red welts on her body. After a long winter, in spring 1887, swarms of mosquitoes began to invade New Iberia once again. To be sure the mosquitoes were a nuisance, but the Wakefields did what they could to keep them away. They rubbed their bodies with repellents made from plants like garlic, and they built fires hoping the smoke would ward them off.

At that time, no one knew that mosquitoes are more than a nuisance. They are also dangerous, carrying deadly diseases like malaria. During Emma's lifetime, malaria was often fatal. It would not be eliminated in the United States until the mid-1900s, when scientists discovered the link between the insects and the disease. Louisiana, with its hot, humid climate and swamps, was a breeding ground for the mosquitoes that carried malaria. From large, heavily populated communities like New Orleans to small, rural communities like New Iberia, malaria affected everyone.

Sadly, when Emma was nineteen years old, her sister Amelia (named after their mother) fell ill with the horrible disease. Emma's mother, undoubtedly, did all she could to save her daughter. It is probable that she brought in doctors to help. She may have even contacted local healers or traiteurs familiar with native herbs and plants. She almost certainly stayed up all night with young Amelia, fighting the disease consuming her. Emma and her siblings witnessed their sister's suffering and their mother's refusal to surrender. Yet the fever would not go down, and chills caused violent shivering. Amelia suffered from vomiting, diarrhea, and pain.

Ultimately, no treatments helped, and young Amelia died. Perhaps her sister's suffering influenced Emma's decision to enter medical school three years later.

WITH TEARS AND TOILING BREATH, FOR AMELIA

What is our sin? Who fails **with**
no intention? **tears**
cloud my vision **and**
evaporate upon my sister's feverish brow, her soul **toiling**
until her last **breath.**

I
struggle to **find**
reason for **thy**
design. Thy **cunning**
diseased **seeds**
plant evil spirits. **O**
woe upon the **million-murdering**
malaria bereaving us of dear Melia, delivering an early **Death.**

The striking line for this golden shovel came from the poem "In Exile" written by Ronald Ross in August 1897. He wrote the poem after his discovery of malaria parasites in *anopheline* mosquitoes. Sir Ross received the Nobel Prize in 1902 for his discovery.

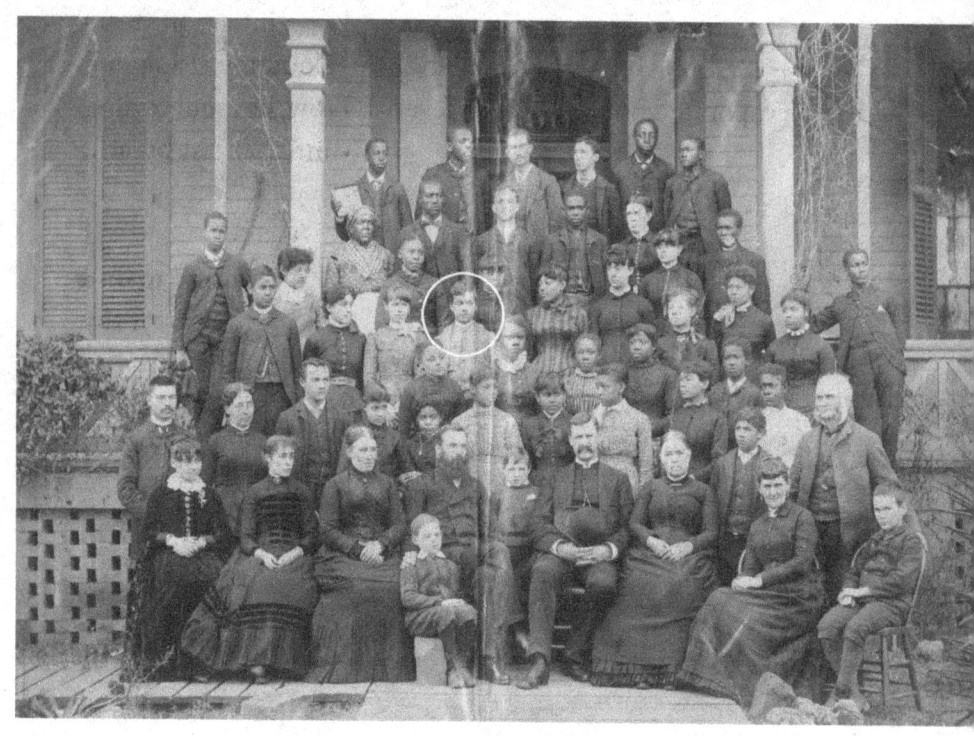

Samuel Wakefield Jr.'s class photo from Straight University. Sammie is center, wearing the light suit (*circled*).

Source: The Historic New Orleans Collection.

1889

ANOTHER TRAGEDY STRIKES

It was cold and cloudy that January day in New Iberia, typical of the weather that time of the year in 1889. At a house on West St. Peter Street, near the intersection with Center Street, a drama was unfolding. More than two hundred White men surrounded the one-and-a-half-story Wakefield family home. They threatened the women inside. Twenty-year-old Emma dared the man pressing the muzzle of his gun to her left breast to pull the trigger:

"Shoot, you dirty dog! Shoot!"

Emma bravely stood with her mother and sisters and demanded that the mob leave their home. They had just shot and killed Sammie, her seventeen-year-old brother, only a few blocks away. Now they wanted her older brother, Adolph, and ransacked the house in an unsuccessful attempt to find him.

Two years after her father's death, Emma's seventeen-year-old brother Samuel Jr., who they called Sammie, was home on break from Straight University. While in town, Sammie shot and killed a twenty-one-year-old White man named James Trainor (sometimes spelled Traynor). According to Sammie's friend, the shooting was in self-defense, but others claimed it was unprovoked. A mob found Sammie and lynched him. The newspapers around town reported different accounts of the murder and lynching.

A Howe Institute[1] teacher, Ms. Capitola L. Robinson, wrote letters to her mother in Akron, Ohio, regarding the lynching of young Samuel. Later, she testified in court about what she saw. She said that she was present when Sammie told his mother and Adolph about the shooting of James Trainer. Ms. Robinson heard Sammie

---

1. The Howe Institute (1888–1933) was one of the earliest schools established for Black students in New Iberia, LA.

say that Trainor assaulted him and used offensive, racist language. Then, Adolph told his brother to go back to work and warned him to not return to the store where Trainor worked. Adolph said that he would take care of things later. Unfortunately, Sammie encountered Trainor on his way back from work. According to Ms. Robinson, Sammie demanded that Trainor apologize. Instead, Trainor tried to assault Sammie again. In response, Sammie pulled out a pistol and shot Trainor, killing him. After the sheriff and his deputy arrested Sammie, a vigilante mob, also known as regulators, formed. They did not want to see Sammie go to prison. They wanted him to die. So, the mob assaulted the sheriff and his deputy, took Sammie, and shot him.

BALLAD FOR SAMMIE

O, what can save me? here I pray,
My brother Sam is dead.
He grabbed a gun while on his way.
Fury was in his head.

Sent on an errand by his boss,
was met by forceful brute;
He walked away, counted a loss,
that White rights would refute.

An argument between two men
has led to angry mobs.
At will, they lynch again, again
ignoring weighty sobs.

Now, here we place his sacred head
Behind the house we stay.
Unearth a grave for heaven's bed;
A curtain veils this day.

As cries of grief fill the air,
I join with bated breath.
For threats to innocents unfair,
Their rage will lead to death.

O, what can save me? here I pray
My brother, Sam, is gone.
Deny my fear for Fear's own way
casts shadows on the dawn.

They Come for Adolph

Two hundred men
surround our house,
Winchester rifles cocked.
Sausage meat! I hear them cry
Come out, Adolph! You're sausage meat!

Brave as a lion, Momma faces the men,
my sister and me by her side.
You cowards, you thieves,
you have no business here.
The son you seek is gone.
Leave us be!

The muzzle of the gun pressing my chest,
I call that White man a dirty dog.
Get away from me with your stinky self;
I dare you to stain my dress!

The prairie black with men and boys fleeing.

We're packing it in,
boarding the train,
leaving this place of sin.

1889

THE WAKEFIELDS LEAVE NEW IBERIA

While still mourning their brother, Emma and her sisters had to return to New Orleans for school. No doubt Emma hugged her mother tightly, kissing her over and over, not wanting to leave her alone in New Iberia. Being the good mother that she was, Amelia insisted that her daughters return to Straight University to complete their education. Their brother Adolph was already there; he would keep the girls safe.

On the day of departure, Emma and her sisters packed their bags and loaded them into a wagon that would take them to the train depot on Jefferson Street. They bid their mother goodbye and then climbed in.

Over the next few years, Amelia would sell the family home on St. Peter Street, as well as other properties the family owned, and join her children in New Orleans. By 1893, the entire Wakefield family had left New Iberia forever.

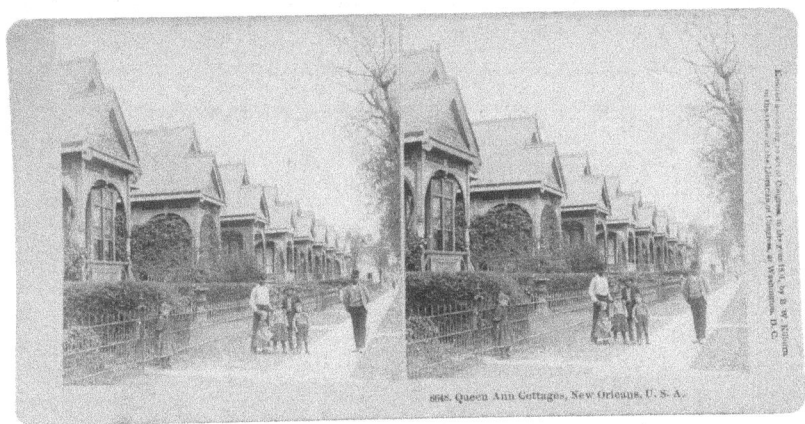

Emma and her family may have lived in homes like these Queen Ann-style cottages in New Orleans after they moved from New Iberia.

Source: Library of Congress Prints and Photographs Division Washington, DC.

1894

Embracing Education

Emma and her siblings embraced their parents' view of education as the vehicle to success. Emma in particular was an exceptional student. She graduated second in her class from Straight University. (Later, she would graduate with honors as a medical student from New Orleans University.)

Because of her hard work, Emma was well prepared for success in any field. She could have become a teacher like her older sister, Mattie, who was one of the first Black teachers in the Iberia Parish public schools. After all, teaching was the popular choice for many young, well-educated African American women of the time.

In addition, with the classical music training she and her siblings received, Emma could have become a concert pianist. Her love for music was so great that she even entertained the idea of delaying the start of her medical practice for a year so she could attend a music conservatory in New York. Although she eventually decided against this idea, Emma nurtured a lifelong passion for music. In 1894, the same year she entered medical school, she performed a piano solo at the school's graduation ceremony.

Emma chose medicine, a field known to be hostile to women and particularly African American women. So, what possessed this brilliant young woman to take this less-traveled path? Her fearlessness and confidence in her ability to complete a degree in medicine was likely nurtured within her family. She witnessed her father's drive for success in business and politics, and then in public service despite many setbacks. And she witnessed her mother's strength and resilience in the face of incredible personal loss. Nothing would prevent her from achieving her goal of becoming a physician.

Fine Oxford Bags for $5.90 to $7.10.

No. 33R5254 Full Shape English Oxford Bag, made up in fine grain leather, heavy riveted frame, leather covered, fine brass spring catches and lock, double handles, leather lined, with pocket on sides. Colors, olive or dark brown.

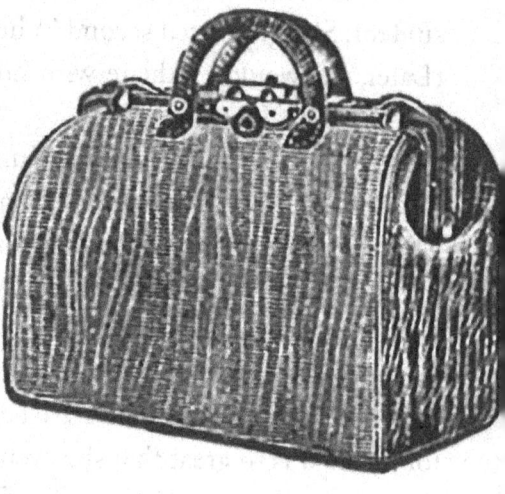

Length	Weight	Price
14 inches	4 lbs.	$5.90
15 inches	4¼ lbs.	6.20
16 inches	4½ lbs.	6.50
17 inches	4¾ lbs.	6.80
18 inches	5 lbs.	7.10

Emma might have carried a bag like this one for her medical tools during school and after she became a physician.

Source: Sears, Roebuck catalog, 1902.

Making a Choice

I have a song that plays inside my head.
I focus on a new melody.

      A melody my heart knew well,
        taken from a high-wire balancing act.

Tones out of balance vibrate from my fingers
with no steady hand to hold me firm.

      Out of balance with no hand to hold,
      I hear echoes of my father's voice.

My father's choice to pay a dollar
for sheet music on a wooden bench.

      Trading a wooden bench for a medical bag
      I carry instruments for a caring future.

I carry instruments for a caring future.
I have a song that plays inside my head.

1897

EMMA BECOMES A PHYSICIAN

Beginning in the early nineteenth century, African American men (such as Dr. James McCune Smith in the 1830s) and women (like Dr. Rebecca Lee Crumpler in 1864) pursued and earned medical degrees. All attended medical schools at White universities in the northern United States or abroad. It was not until 1868 that Howard University opened the nation's first medical department for African Americans. It took more than twenty years for Louisiana to get its own such program.

Even though Black students began receiving medical training, at that time very few hospitals would hire them, especially hospitals with White patients. Moreover, most of the hospitals in the city refused to treat African Americans. So, the New Orleans chapter of a charity organization known as the Phillis Wheatley Club worked to create a hospital specifically for Black patients. In 1896, they established the Phillis Wheatley Sanatorium and Training School for Nurses to address the medical needs of the African American community in New Orleans. It also provided training opportunities for nurses, medical students, and professionals.

Unfortunately, despite the club's good intentions, the hospital soon struggled to make enough money to stay open. Thankfully, they found help from two sources. New Orleans University had been founded in 1869 for African American students, much like many other historically Black colleges and universities (HBCUs) around the country. The university agreed to make the sanatorium part of their medical school. Second, a wealthy donor named John D. Flint of Massachusetts agreed to give money to the school to fund the medical program and hospital. In his honor, the medical school was renamed Flint Medical College. The hospital was moved to a new location on Canal Street and renamed the Flint-Goodridge Hospital.

From the beginning, it attracted the finest candidates through its rigorous program.

Emma Wakefield entered New Orleans University's medical school at just the right time. In 1894, while the Phillis Wheatley Club was working to create the new hospital, the state legislature passed a law that allowed women admission to Louisiana medical schools. Shortly after that, the New Orleans University Medical Department admitted three young women. Twenty-four-year-old Emma was one of the three. How exciting it must have been for Emma and her classmates to be among the first to actually use the new training facility! The hospital provided them with the clinical and surgical training that prepared them for excellence as medical professionals. Surely, Emma and her classmates benefited greatly from the training they received at the new hospital.

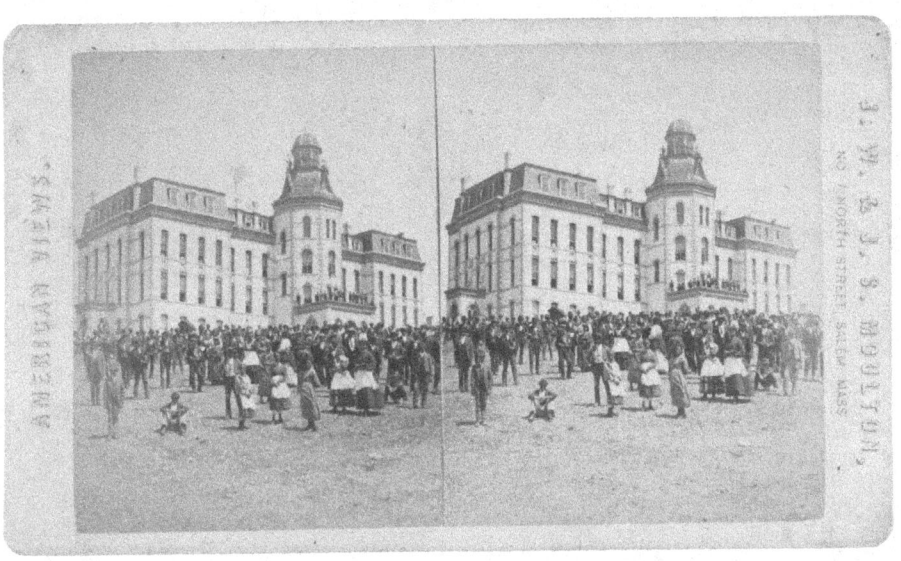

In the 1800s, many people enjoyed viewing stereographs, or two photographs side-by-side. When viewed together through a stereoscope, the images formed one three-dimensional picture. This stereograph shows a crowd of African American students on the lawn of Howard University, in Washington, DC. Like New Orleans University, Howard University was founded specifically to educate Black students.

Source: Salem, Mass. : J. W. & J. S. Moulton, Publishers [between 1867 and 1920], Library of Congress.

Phillis Wheatley Club

Phillis Wheatley knew the struggles of slavery,
yet she held a brave pen.
We honor her devotion to words and learning
by forming this club in her name.

With my friend Sylvania, I join efforts
to establish a training hospital.
We welcome women of color
who long to heal others

with loving care. We seek to be bold,
to serve, and belong. I offer my medical
experience as much as I am able
between lab days and studying nights.

Supplies are few; we struggle to secure funding,
yet in a spirit of holding up
women of our race to a higher standard,
we stand beside men; we show them what we know.

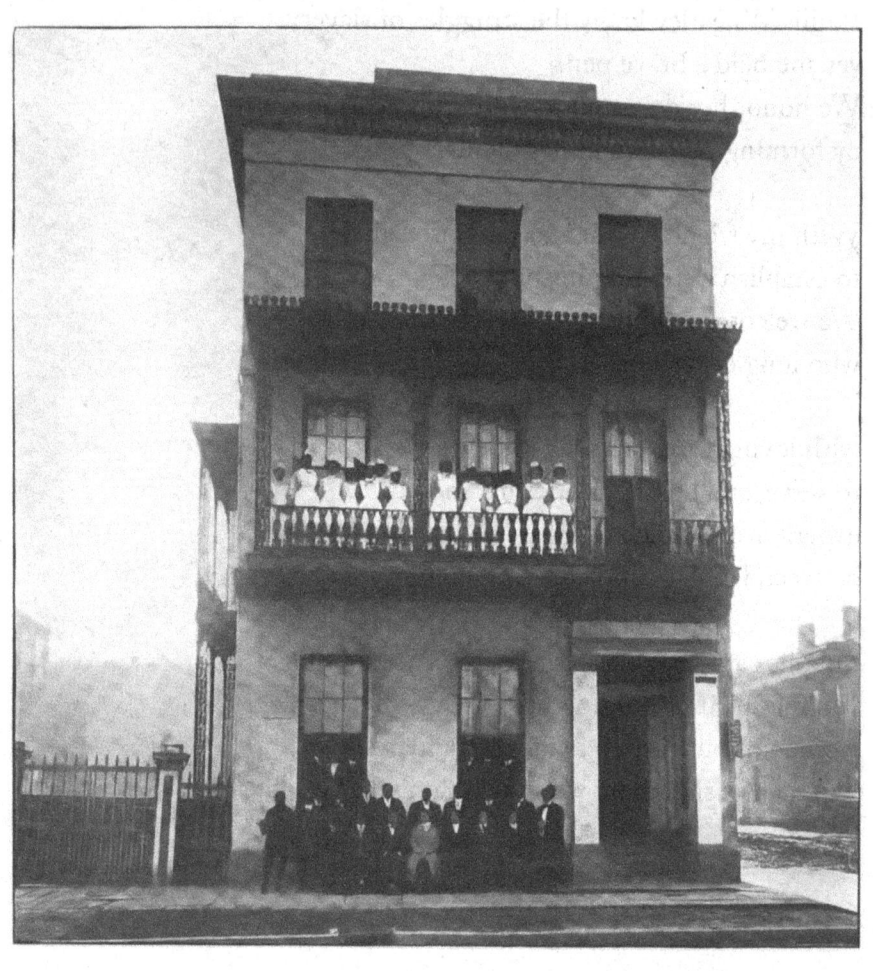

Flint-Goodridge Hospital, Canal Street, New Orleans, 1916.

Source: Xavier University Library Archives.

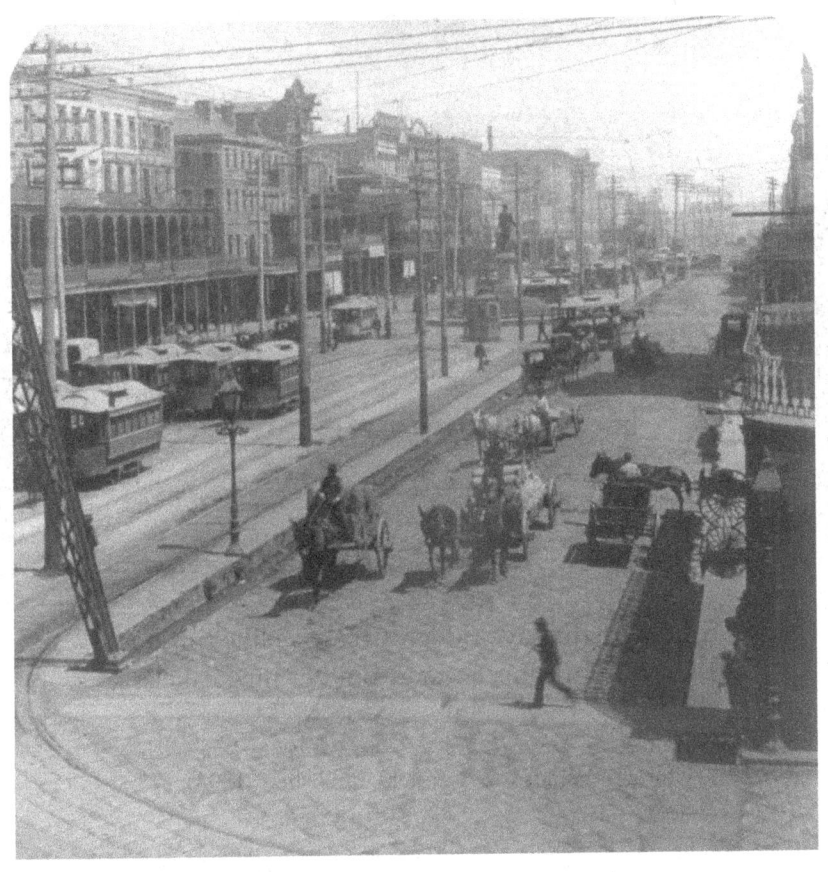

This photograph of Canal Street was taken around 1891, just a few years before Emma Wakefield would begin her medical courses in New Orleans. The Flint-Goodridge Hospital where she trained was located on this street.

Source: Washington, DC: J. F. Jarvis, Publisher, c. June 2, 1891.
Courtesy of the Library of Congress.

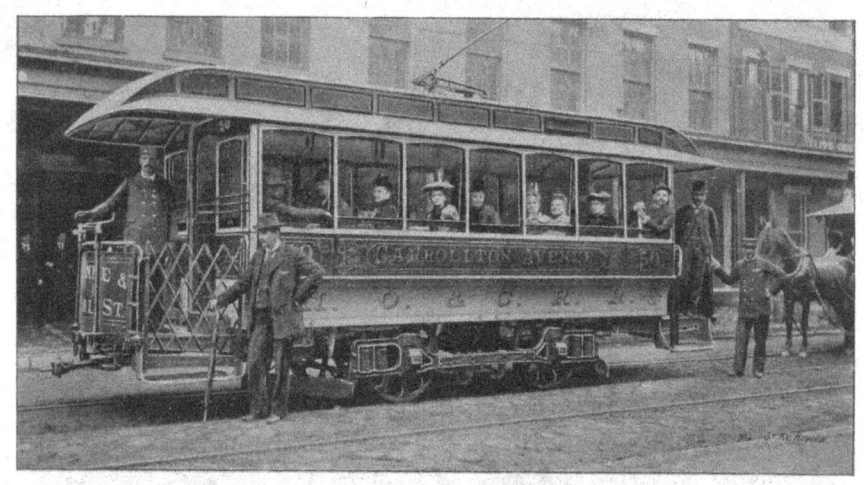

Emma might have ridden streetcars like this one, the Carrollton Line, to and from her medical classes.

Source: *The Street Railway Review: Index to Volume III* (Chicago: Windsor & Kenfield, Publishers, 1893), 173.

Riding Home on the Streetcar

After a long clinical day, the streetcar fills up—
sanctioned to the back
coal-colored workers from the lumber yard,
nurses with blood-splattered shoes,
and me, weary and withering.

Through glassless window frames,
a light breeze softens the stale air.
Mule snuffs, brays, lumbers on, pulling its heavy load.
The Basin Canal glistens, reflecting shadows
of sails lowering like the western sun.

My body knows tired.
It slumps into the wooden-slatted seat
gathering strength
for the mile walk home.

1897

"Exceptionally Excellent" Emma

By graduation in 1897, Emma was the only woman remaining in the program. She graduated with honors and went on to distinguish herself further by her excellent performance on the state's medical licensure examination. She could have justified quitting medical school when the other two young women dropped out, but she did not. The resilient spirit that had been kindled within her would not let her quit. Emma was determined to be a physician.

It is probable that Emma was inspired by the story of Dr. Rebecca Lee Crumpler. Dr. Crumpler became the first Black woman in the United States to graduate with a medical degree in 1864. As a trailblazer, Dr. Crumpler's accomplishments must have gone far in inspiring young women like Emma to dream of a career in medicine. In addition, Emma almost certainly would have known of Dr. Elizabeth Magnus Cohen, the New Yorker who was Louisiana's first woman physician. Dr. Cohen lived in the French Quarter at the same time Emma and her family lived there. What is more, Emma received much attention from the newspapers when she graduated medical school and again when she performed so well on the state medical examination. It is very likely that Dr. Cohen, one of Emma's possible role models, had heard of Emma as well. Emma established her own medical practice in New Orleans and advertised her hours in the newspaper.

DR. EMMA WAKEFIELD.

Her Exceptionally Excellent Examination Before the State Board.

Dr. Emma Wakefield, who passed the State Board of Medical Examiners last week with honors, and submitted one of the best papers passed upon by the board, is a native of this State, a daughter of the late Samuel Wakefield, State Senator from New Iberia, and at one time deputy naval officer at this port. She is about twenty-six years of age, pretty, intelligent and well educated. She matriculated at the New Orleans Medical College four years ago with two other young friends. Of the latter, one left the same year to engage in teaching; she is now, however, pursuing a literary course in Boston; the other, two years after, married and left the college. Dr. Wakefield, although the only female student left in the institution, persisted in her studies. She worked diligently and made a splendid record in all the branches of the school. She proved one of the best students in her class, as her examination before the State board proves.

Dr. Wakefield is not the first colored woman physician in America, several others having graduated from Northern and Western colleges, but she is the first woman who studied medicine and received the degree of M. D. in Louisiana and the South, or at least in the Gulf States.

Dr. Wakefield is also accomplished as a musician, being an excellent performer on the piano. She is undecided as to whether she will settle down to practice at once or to go North and spend a year in a conservatory; but when she does make up her mind to begin practice she will probably make diseases of children a specialty. Dr. Wakefield lives in the French quarter with her mother and two sisters. She has another sister, a widow, who also resides in this city, and who held a position in the United States Mint for several years, and a brother, Adolphe J. Wakefield, who is in business in Houston, Tex.

Emma performed so well on her medical exam—and because she was the first woman of any race to earn a medical degree in Louisiana—that it was reported in the local newspaper.

Source: New Orleans *Times-Democrat*, April 20, 1897.

Graduation Sestina

The sheepskin in my hand
feels soft and light,
a scroll engraved with years
of focused eyes
on microscopic cells searching for answers
to epidemics, diseases, and fevers.

Jenner and Pasteur found cures for the fevers
softening my medico hand
with practical, thoughtful answers.
Today, physicians are light
to dark unsanitary conditions. We've seen eyes
of suffering for too many years.

No more saddlebags of useless cures or unclean years.
No more smallpox, malaria, and scarlet fever.
We've opened our eyes
to science of nature, a broader hand
on the pulse of cells has come to light.
As physicians, we are called to find answers.

To have full advantage of these answers
as we embark on a career for future years.
Turn of the century will beam a light
on the future of medicine, no fever
will go untouched by our collective hand.
These seven men graduate with me, and our eyes

will meet the gaze of thousands of eyes
searching for healing answers.
We offer our ready and willing hand
to the epidemic years.

Can you feel my fever
to put into practice my expertise? The light

of my knowledge will light
up the grief in their eyes.
I will cure your fever.
I will find the answers
to soften the blow from enslaved years.
My hand is a gentle, wise hand.

Advertisement: Have a fever? Dr. Wakefield's light
and gentle hand will open your eyes
to understand the answers to many healthy years.

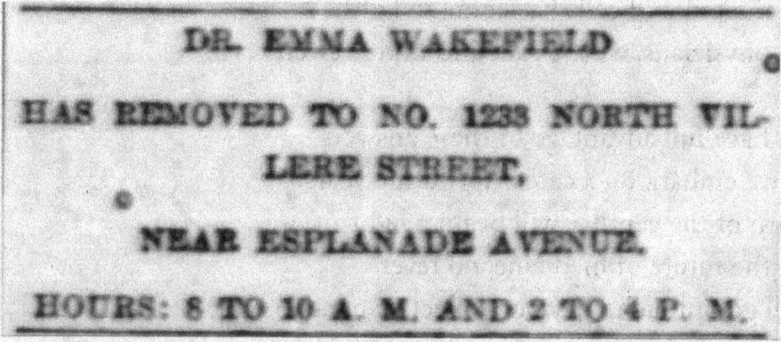

After graduation, Emma set up her own medical practice in New Orleans. She announced the new office location and hours in the New Orleans *Times-Democrat* on July 3, 1898.

Some People Say

Some people say it's a miracle of modern times,
When they consider the walls I've climbed.

A woman, a doctor?
A woman of color, a doctor?

Some people say
moral degradation
emerges from a slave nation.

Some people say
mental prowess
is not for the lowest.

But I say
my mind is a marvelous
gift from God

I say my heart grows
with yearning to bless.

My zeal is conceived to elevate.

I am the new hero,
a valiant servant to my race.

I seek no charity.

I knock at the door of Justice.
and burst through in Glory.

Inspiration for this poem came from "The Progress of Colored Women," a speech given in 1904 by Mary Church Terrell, 1896 president of the National Association of Colored Women.

1899

THE WAKEFIELDS LEAVE LOUISIANA

A few years after Emma graduated, she and her entire family packed up their belongings and boarded a steam train for San Francisco, California. In Louisiana, racial tensions had risen in the years after Reconstruction. For example, the state's Separate Car Act forced people of African American heritage to sit in a separate, Blacks-only railcar. In 1891, Homer Plessy, a Creole of color who was often mistaken for White, decided to test the law by sitting in the Whites-only railcar. When the conductor told Plessy to move to the other car, he refused. As an American citizen, he said, he had the freedom to sit anywhere he wanted. Because he would not move, he was arrested. In the end, the Supreme Court upheld the law, stating that different facilities for the races were constitutional so long as they were "separate but equal."

Like Homer Plessy, who was only one-eighth Black, Emma was a fair African American. Yet she still experienced much discrimination. Perhaps the oppression of the time pushed her family to leave Louisiana. News of greater opportunities for African Americans in other states could have led them to dream of a new life beyond the South. Neither Emma nor her other family members left any records explaining why they left Louisiana.

Yet once they arrived in California, they had another reason to celebrate: Emma married Joseph Oscar Paillet on January 10, 1900. Her new husband was also a Louisiana native, the son of Hillaire and Elodie Lemelle Paillet of Opelousas. Over the course of their marriage, Joseph held various skilled labor jobs, including wagon maker, drayman (someone who hauls goods by dray, a kind of cart), and blacksmith.

Now that she was in California, Emma would have to get a new medical license from the California Board of Medical Examiners. Even though she had already passed the exam in Louisiana, she would have to prove herself again in the new state. While awaiting her medical license, Emma relied on her musical training and taught piano lessons. One New Orleans newspaper wrote that she attended the Grand Conservatory of Music to continue her piano training. In the 1900 Census—the government's official count of all the citizens in the country—she was listed as a music teacher, not a doctor.

A year later, in 1901, the California State Medical Board issued Emma a license to practice medicine in the state. This meant she could resume her medical practice.

Riding the Train in the Dark

If I sit in the colored car
on the train to New Orleans
am I approving the Jim Crow laws?

Would I dare sit next to Homer Plessy
in the "all White" section
and protest separate cars?
If the conductor asks me my color,
would I say Black or White?
Who knows the truth?
What court of Supreme Rule
agrees to separation
after a Civil War for freedom?
In this day, with African blood
in my veins, can I pursue
a dream?
How can I become who I am meant to be
when every "For Whites Only" chair
is covered in fake
upholstery of fairness?
Justice Henry Billings Brown would have us believe
we choose this plight,
choose to be inferior.
Would anyone choose
separate over equal?
Colored car over White car?

Ode to the Steam Locomotive: 1900

As I embark upon the Main Line of Mid-America,
I praise this locomotive, its rising steam,
its speed and force
to take me far from here—North:

Oh, simmering cauldrons
your steam aspires
to gathering clouds
waving wind with fire.
Piston pressing through iron walls
drives quick movement forward.

Oh, giant of steel
wield your large limbs,
shake the good earth.
From flame to sparkling ore,
smoke rises to lead-lined towers
and breathes like a majestic dragon.

Oh, vast wheels whirl
trembling force fingers twirl
past fields of golden wheat
through snow-capped mountainsides.

I ride
hand in Joseph's hand
our flying chariot
to future air.

Wedding Eintou

Circle
my wedding ring
glows wisdom found in love
repeated vows forever worn
committing two of us
life together
I do

1900

"Passing for White"

Interestingly, much of the information on Emma and her family in that 1900 Census is incorrect. For example, Emma is listed as thirty years old and married for five years. Moreover, the census form lists her place of birth as Cuba. Emma's mother's name is misspelled (Emilia), and she is listed as having five children, all alive at the time of the census. In fact, Amelia had given birth to seven children, and by the 1900 Census two had died. Perhaps this inaccurate information is due to a miscommunication between the Wakefields and the census taker. Sometimes, people did not give the census takers honest answers, thinking people asking questions might be tax collectors or other agents trying to trick them. Or it could be a copying error, as all the many census documents were combined into one.

The census form raises another question about Emma's life in California. Despite giving her race as Black in that census, after 1900, California civil records mark Emma and her family's race as White. Whether the Wakefields intentionally passed for White is unknown.

"Passing for White" was a common practice among many fair-complexioned, mixed-race African Americans. On official government forms, they changed their race from "Negro," "Black," "Colored," "Mulatto," or "Mixed" to "White." In this way, they escaped the racism and discrimination they experienced as African Americans and took advantage of opportunities available to Whites only. This meant better treatment, jobs, education, health care, housing, and so on.

Passing for White, or *"passé blanc"* as it was known in Louisiana, was especially popular among Afro-Creole families of New Orleans and south Louisiana. Members of such communities had both European and African ancestors. However, when these Creoles left Louisiana and settled in other parts of the country or world, many chose to identify as White or Caucasian.

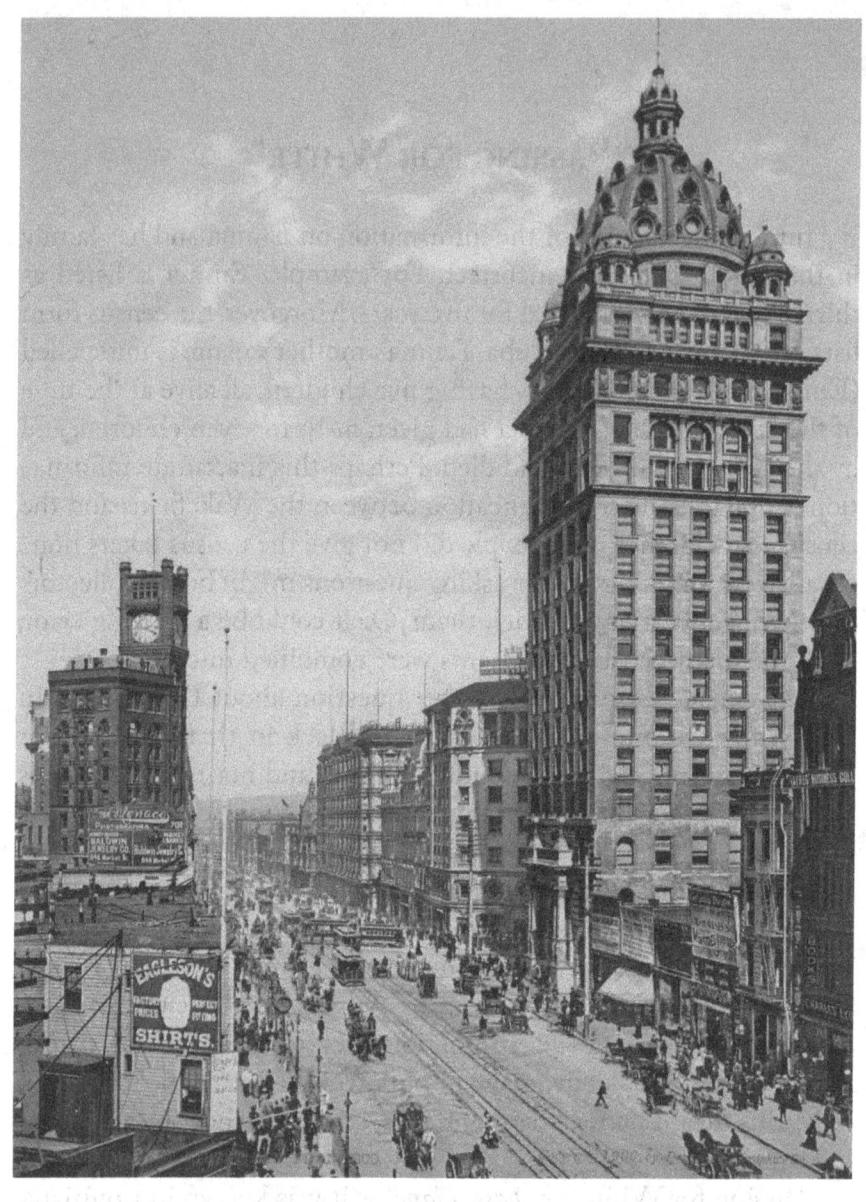

Market Street in San Francisco, 1900.

Source: Library of Congress Prints and Photographs Division, Washington, DC.

SAN FRANCISCO, 1901

San Francisco welcomes me
sending a beam of sunshine
over bay fog.

No one knows where I've been.
No one sees brown dirt on my feet.
No one knows my grief or shame.

I look into every face
expecting eyes of hatred.
I check every wrist
for the pulse of prejudice.

They don't see my color.
I am simply their doctor.

Hello, Dr. Paillet, *Good day*.
Good day.

1902

ANOTHER SISTER LOST

The future seemed promising for Emma: she had just married, and she was now a practicing physician. Yet within two years of moving to San Francisco, tragedy would strike once again. Emma lost two more siblings within one month of each other: Mary Victoria (June 10, 1902) and Adolph (July 16, 1902).

Victoria was only twenty-five years old and living with Emma and her husband when she died. Not much is known about Victoria's life in San Francisco. She suffered a sudden epileptic seizure, which sadly took her life.

Funeral records say that the family had a history of epilepsy, including her father and brother. Though the records do not say which brother may have suffered from the condition, it was likely Sammie. Adolph, a successful officer in the Spanish-American War, probably would have been prevented from enlisting with such a medical history.

INVICTUS

I am the master of my fate:
I am the captain of my soul.
   —William Ernest Henley

Out of the grief that burdens me,
      Dark as the night without a moon,
I thank poets of history
      For setting down my endless tune.

In wake of Victoria's song,
      Her heart too young to overcome.
Under these losses, I am strong.
      My head is bowed; I won't succumb.

Beyond the seizures of her time
      Awaits a cure I long to find,
And I honor her life sublime,
      My heart beats strength into my mind.

It matters not how steep or wide,
      How charged the epileptic toll,
I am a rower on the tide:
      I am the sower of my soul.

Inspired by "Invictus," an often-quoted poem written by William Ernest Henry, a British poet, in 1875. *Invictus* is a Latin word that means unconquered.

1902

Cholera Claims Adolph Wakefield

After their father Samuel died in 1883, the Wakefields' eldest son, Adolph, stepped into his father's shoes. He took on the role of head of the family. Even though Adolph was only twenty-three years old at the time, he was in many ways like his father. By the time his father passed, Adolph had graduated from Straight University and established his own businesses. He had earned various positions at the Custom House in New Orleans and, like his father, served as a colored commissioner for the Iberia Parish school system. One year later, he was elected clerk of court for Iberia Parish. To Emma and her family, Adolph was more than a businessman, politician, and public servant. He was their provider and protector.

Emma viewed Adolph as a hero. But she was not alone. In 1898, the United States entered the Spanish-American War, both to help Cuba fight for independence from Spain and take over other Spanish territories. President McKinley soon allowed Black men to serve in the military. The president's advisers convinced him that it would be prudent to allow Black men to enlist and form their own regiments. It was commonly, though wrongly, believed at the time that Black people were immune to tropical diseases known to thrive in Cuba and other island nations. Adolph joined the United States Volunteer Infantry (USVI), Company I, Ninth Regiment. The Ninth Regiment, a mounted regiment (one that rode on horseback), was one of the few created for African American soldiers. Adolph's regiment later received praise from the US government for the courage, discipline, and horsemanship of its men.

Adolph quickly rose through the ranks, ultimately achieving the rank of first lieutenant in recognition of his bravery and leadership. In 1899, when one of his privates was murdered by Cuban bandits, Adolph and his men hunted them down. They engaged in a fierce battle with the bandits and won. His superior officers wrote, "He

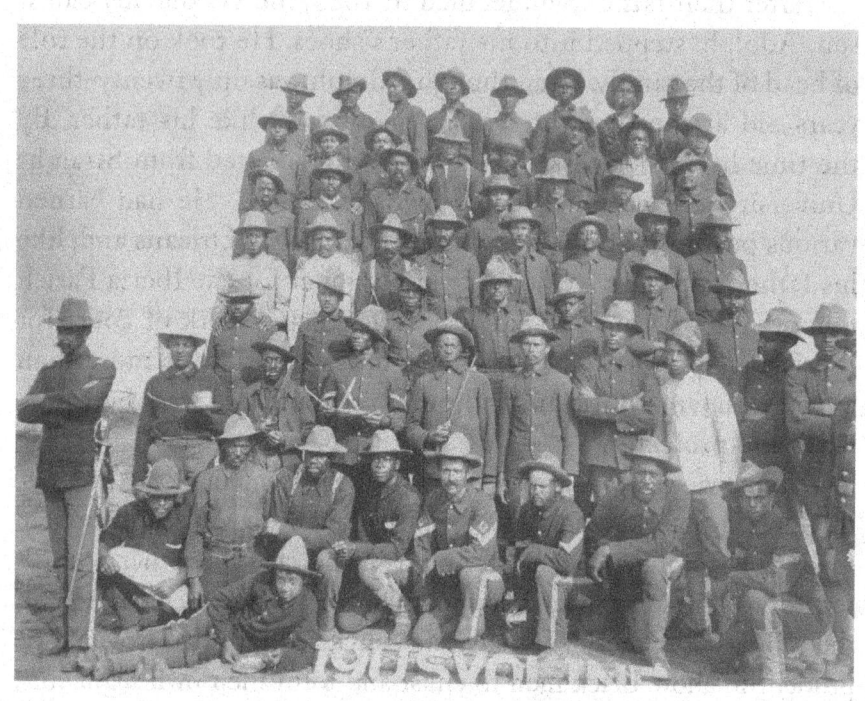

When Adolph enlisted in the US Army, he joined the Volunteer Infantry, Company I, Ninth Regiment. This photograph of the company was taken in 1899. It is unknown if Adolph is included here.

Source: Photograph by L. Leland Barton, courtesy of the Library of Congress.

showed great courage in fighting in San Ana," and was believed "to be of heroic mould."

When Adolph told his family of his intention to fight in the Spanish-American War, Emma surely feared for his safety and that of his comrades. As a physician, she likely knew that his race would not protect him from the tropical diseases that sickened and killed so many American soldiers of every race. Emma also would have known that his race would not protect him from the bullets and bayonets aimed in his direction.

The Spanish-American War ended in 1898 with a victory for the United States. As a result, Spanish territories like the Philippines, Guam, and Puerto Rico became American territories. Shortly after returning home from the war, Adolph was again sent away, this time to serve in the Philippines. Like the Cubans, the people of the Philippines wanted independence. But the islands provided a major port for trade in Asia, and the United States was not ready to lose it. The US Army was sent there to put down what it saw as a rebellion.

Soon, Adolph began showing signs of illness known as cholera. Cholera is an often-deadly disease passed through unsafe food and water. Sadly, in July 1902, while still in the Philippines, Adolph died at the age of forty-two. Mamie Wakefield, Adolph's widow, applied to receive his pension, funds set aside by the government for Adolph when he was done with his military service. Pensions provide money for a person to live on after they have left a job, as thanks for their hard work. However, the US Army claimed that Adolph had not gotten sick during his active duty, and so her appeal for his pension was denied.

Mrs. Mamie Wakefield filled out this form to request a widow's pension. The claim was denied by the US Army.

Source: National Archives, Widow Pension Record.

Thirteen Ways of Looking at Cholera

I
When duty calls,
being the good and noble
man, Adolph goes.

II
In a war, no one
worries about cleanliness.
Mud and muck are all part of it.

III
Side by side, Black
or White
soldiers shoulder the burden
together.

IV
Where is the water?
Water, Water,
thirst unquenched.

V
He is dirty,
black and blue face,
disparity of race.

VI
Hand to hand
supply clerk in the Philippines
hands *Vibrio Cholera*
contamination
to my brother.

VII
Adolph is one
 of 200,000—
epidemic score.

VIII
The skin dies first
as rice-water
leaks on and on.

IX
A hero works through
stomach pains. Doesn't foresee
the light of God.

X
Far from home,
we could pretend
it doesn't affect us.

XI
My brother dies
alone
far away
buried,
lost,
gone.

XII
To avoid infection,
wash your hands,
like the Army
washed its hands
of responsibility.

XIII
Mamie becomes a widow
with no pension check.
Casualties of war
are never fair.

> **DR. EMMA WAKEFIELD-PAILLET RETURNS AFTER SEVEN YEARS.**
>
> After an absence of seven years on the Pacific Coast, Dr. Paillet has returned to New Orleans to remain permanently. The doctor, although known in musical circles here, will be especially remembered as the first woman in the Gulf States to graduate in medicine. While in San Francisco she perfected her musical education under the most competent teachers. She spent two years at the Grand Conservatory of Music and one year under San Francisco's most eminent technician, Prof. Hugo Mansfeldt, who gave her every encouragement to become a great pianiste. As music has always been the doctor's chosen profession, she is undecided whether to resume the practice of medicine in the Crescent City or establish herself as a teacher of piano technic.

A New Orleans newspaper announced Emma's return to the city. Clearly, she was known so well around the city that her return to Louisiana was worth printing in the newspaper.

Source: New Orleans *Times-Democrat*, September 16, 1906.

1906

Returning to Louisiana

Emma left few records of those years in California and her siblings' deaths. Hopefully she spent quality time with her remaining family members and took pride in her medical practice. Nevertheless, it would not be long before the Wakefields were on the move again. Emma's mother returned to New Orleans sometime before 1905. Two years later, on February 15, 1907, at age sixty-nine, Amelia died. Before her passing, she had moved into the Thomy Lafon Old Folks' Home, a nursing home on Rampart Street, perhaps so as not to burden her children with her care.

The year after Amelia's death, the records from Straight University show that Emma and her husband were both living in one of the residence halls on campus. Additionally, in the 1908 city directory, Emma is listed as a physician. This suggests that she was in Louisiana long enough to reopen her medical practice.

Once again, Emma left no answers as to why she and her husband left California. It may be that the destructive 1906 San Francisco earthquake forced her and Joseph to flee the city. Or perhaps they returned to New Orleans so Emma could care for her mother and settle her affairs. Whatever the reason for her return to New Orleans, Dr. Emma Wakefield-Paillet was back in New Orleans practicing medicine.

Sonnet After the San Francisco Earthquake, 1906

On ground that shakes where displaced people tread,
In shattered homes where flames endanger them,
I care for bones and nerves. I serve them bread.
From heart to hand, our might will overcome.

When I forgive the tragedies I've known,
I look not on the troubles of my past,
and move to make allegiance of my own.
Are loads too heavy for my strength to last?

As loss of leaves from oaks, my family tree
my father, brothers, sisters all are gone,
I beg to know who I'm supposed to be
and why I am the one who must go on.

In giving I am living. Still I roam:
That longing search for place to call my home.

Today I Will Praise

Today I will praise love—
>how a mother loves
>unconditionally.

I will praise her tireless heart
Praise the way it bore
>the pain of loss,
>>husband, sons, daughters.

Praise her lift to the wings
I fly on—Praise her gentle catch
when I fall.
>I will open my hands in adoration
>of how her burdens so heavy
>could seem so light.

I will praise migration that led
her north to me.

Praise the northwest
>for acceptance and hope.

Praise the rising sun. How she loved the scent of rain.

Praise the gift of my name.
>How it passed from her lips like a hum.

I will praise her hands.
Praise the cradle of them
>holding me, me holding her.

Praise the breath of life.

Praise the Crescent City
      that wrapped her in humid heat
      buried her in sainted stone.

Inspired by Angelo "Eyeambic" Geter, a modern spoken-word poet. His poem "Praise" appears on Grateful.org.

1946

THE END OF EMMA'S LIFE

Eventually, Emma and Joseph returned to California, where they lived the remainder of their lives. For a time, they lived in San Francisco. While there, all their official documents listed the couple as White, not Black. It seems they decided to pass for White when they returned to the state, though they left no explanation for this decision. Sadly, after thirty-five years of marriage, Joseph passed away on May 2, 1935.

After Joseph's death, Emma moved to Oakland, California. There, she rented a house and took a roommate, named Delia Dabbs. Like Emma, Delia was a widow. Perhaps Delia helped Emma cope with the loneliness after her husband's passing. Five years later, in the 1940 Census, Emma is listed once more as Black. As she got older, maybe Emma decided to reclaim her race and heritage.

Finally, on August 26, 1946, at seventy-eight years old, Emma Wakefield-Paillet passed away. She was buried in San Francisco.

Though Emma and Joseph never had children, she certainly left a legacy both in Louisiana and around the country. Newspapers across the United States announced when she passed the Louisiana medical examination. No doubt many women, especially women of color, were inspired by Emma's achievement. Nearly seventy years after Emma's passing, the Iberia African American Historical Society began a campaign to honor her. On November 3, 2018, the town of New Iberia placed a historical marker in front of the central Bouligny Plaza to commemorate Emma's life, including her hard work, her resilience, and her remarkable trail-blazing in the field of medicine.

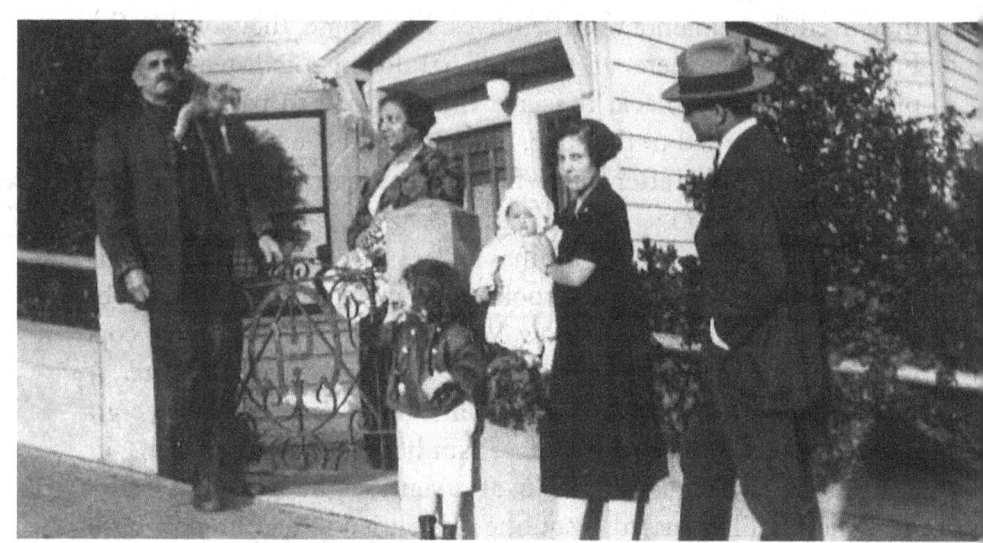

This 1925 picture shows Emma Wakefield-Paillet (*second from left*) and her husband, Joseph (*holding the cat*), visiting with relatives in San Francisco.

Source: Courtesy of Kristin Amundsen, Joseph Paillet's niece.

I Know Who I Am

I know who I am.
I was born during Reconstruction
in newly formed Iberia Parish.
I know about growing up on the bayou.
I know about enslaved sacrifices.
I know education is survival.
I know all these things about myself.

I know what I care about.
I know I care about the body:
how it works,
how it heals,
how it lives.
I know I reject White vigilantes: They,
in their hatred,
trespass, terrorize,
and discard dignity.

I know not all Whites are evil.
I know not all Blacks are kind.
I know why my work is important.
I speak love.
I hold new life in my hands.
I rise.
I know who I am.

Inspired by Ernest Gaines, *Voices from Louisiana* edited by Ann Brewster Dobie, LSU Press, 2018.

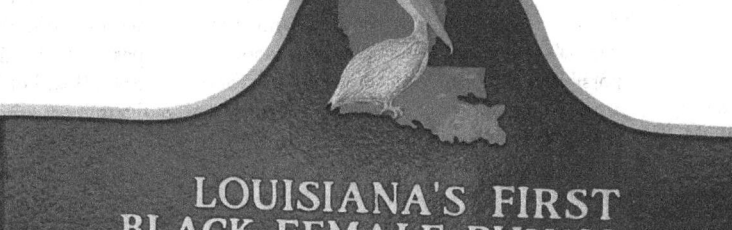

Historical marker placed in downtown New Iberia, Bouligny Plaza, by the Iberia African American Historical Society in 2018. Photo courtesy of the authors.

Timeline of Emma Wakefield-Paillet's Life

November 21, 1868
Emma is born, the fourth child to Samuel and Amelia Valentine Wakefield.

1883
Emma's father dies, possibly by suicide, at the home of his sister, Mary Alice, and brother-in-law, Henderson Ford.

1889
Emma's younger brother, Samuel Jr., is lynched (shot) in New Iberia for killing a twenty-one-year-old White man named James Trainor (Traynor).

April 15, 1897
Emma graduates from her medical program with honors. She passes the Louisiana State Board of Medical Examiners exam with high distinction. She is the only female candidate.

1874–76
Samuel Wakefield serves in the state senate.

1887
Emma's sister, Amelia, dies in New Iberia from malaria.

1894
The Louisiana legislature allows state medical schools and colleges to admit women for the first time. Emma and two other young women immediately enroll in the Medical Department of New Orleans University.

1898–99
Adolph Wakefield is appointed first lieutenant of the volunteer infantry for New Orleans, sent to Cuba.

1899
Emma and her family move to San Francisco, California.

1901
Emma receives her medical license from the state of California, and she begins to practice medicine in San Francisco.

1906
A massive earthquake rocks San Francisco.

Emma and her husband return to New Orleans, and she resumes her New Orleans medical practice.

Date unknown
Emma and Joseph return to San Francisco.

August 26, 1946
Emma dies at age seventy-eight. She is buried in San Francisco.

January 10, 1900
Emma marries Joseph Oscar Paillet, son of Hilaire and Elodie Lemelle Paillet of Opelousas, Louisiana, in San Francisco, California.

1902
Mary Victoria, Emma's sister, dies from epilepsy.

Adolph succumbs to cholera.

1907
Emma's mother dies in New Orleans.

May 2, 1935
Joseph Oscar Paillet dies. He is buried in San Francisco.

Historical Background

Louisiana's first woman physician of African descent just barely missed being born into slavery. Emma's parents and three older siblings were all enslaved. By the time Emma came along in 1868, slavery in New Iberia had been abolished. Yet before the Civil War, slavery had been common practice since before the United States declared independence. In fact, slavery was at the core of the Antebellum Period, which extended from the end of the War of 1812 to the start of the Civil War in 1861. The term "antebellum" means "before war."

In the Antebellum Period, the economy of the South was almost completely dependent on farming. In order to increase their crops, as well as their profits, large landowners relied on forced human labor. They could demand, through violence, that enslaved people work for hours without stopping, under terrible conditions. What's more, plantation owners did not have to pay for the labor, which meant greater profits. They used these profits to buy up more land, as well as more enslaved people. They grew incredibly wealthy. Northern states, by contrast, relied mainly on trade and manufacturing for their economy.

A Life of Enslavement

Slavery was a horrific system. Men, women, and children were forced to work under appalling conditions and endure torture such as lashings and brandings. Most were forced to work from sunup to sundown, often with inadequate food, shelter, and clothing. Enslaved people were viewed as less than human and, as such, had no legal rights. At any time, family members could be sold away from each other, with little hope of ever seeing loved ones again.

When slaveholders died, any enslaved people they held would be listed as their property, or what's known as probate inventory. Probate inventory included furniture, silverware, dishes, real estate, farm animals, and even human beings. Enslaved people were typically listed by name, age, skin color, value, and occasionally other descriptors, such as the status of their health.

South Louisiana records were often written in French as well as English (and sometimes in Spanish). The language used reflected the country that governed Louisiana at the time the record was created. For example, a sale document created when Louisiana was a Spanish territory included the following line: "*Simon, 18 anos, mulato, 250 piastres*" (translation: "Simon, 18 years, mulatto, 250 piastres"). The term "mulatto" is an old (and offensive) term used to identify a person as "mixed-race," usually due to having one Black parent and one White parent.

Later, when the Louisiana territory changed hands and France took over, civil records were written in French: "*James, vingt ans, negre, 900 dollars*" (translation: "James, 20 years, Negro, 900 dollars"). Sale documents listed the person being sold as a "slave for life." Being a "slave for life," in general, meant that one was doomed to be enslaved forever. It also meant that one's children, grandchildren, great-grandchildren, and so on were doomed to be enslaved.

However, Louisiana's unique laws gave slaveholders the power to "manumit" or free their enslaved laborers under certain conditions. Enslaved people could be freed as reward for "good and faithful service" or if they were related to their enslavers. Many enslaved people were closely related to slaveholders, as either their children or their siblings. Under Louisiana law, enslaved people could also purchase their own freedom or that of their family members, if the slaveholder agreed. Formerly enslaved people became known as "free people of color." They had the joy of knowing that all of their descendants would be born free. Most southern states did not have manumission laws like Louisiana's. This meant that the territory (and later, the US state) had a significant population of free people of color.

In some cases, enslaved people fought back by escaping from the sites of their enslavement. Sometimes, abolitionist groups were able to help them travel in secret to the North, where they could be free. Many were captured and returned to their enslavers, but some were able to escape.

Nineteenth-century New Iberia's economy relied firmly on sugarcane. The lifespans of enslaved people on Louisiana sugarcane plantations were extremely short. Threats to life and limb were everywhere on such plantations. Danger lurked in the planting and maintenance of the cane in the extreme Louisiana heat, as well as in the processing of the crop after harvesting. After bringing the cane to the mills, enslaved workers often became victims of horrible accidents during the grinding of the cane and boiling of the cane juice in the huge black sugar kettles. During harvesting seasons, enslaved people worked extremely long hours, seven days a week. Fatigue often made them vulnerable to accidents as well.

To understand how important enslaved people were to the creation of wealth for the sugar planters, one can look at the Weeks family inventory of New Iberia. In 1836, William Weeks held 360 men, women, and children in slavery on his two plantations (Grand Côte and the Shadows of New Iberia). At the time, Weeks's estate was valued at $157,745. In today's currency, his estate would be worth millions of dollars.

A Nation Divided

Over time, the abolitionist movement began to grow, especially in northern states. Abolitionists believed that slavery was wrong and wanted to see it ended throughout the country. In response, southern politicians fought to protect the economic interests of their slaveholding states. Then, Abraham Lincoln was elected president in 1860. Lincoln had said that if he won, he would not eliminate slavery in the South. But he did want to prevent any new US territories from allowing forced labor. His election was a signal that southern states had lost their influence in Congress. They would rather go to war than lose their wealth and way of life.

Most historians agree that the main cause of the Civil War was slavery. Fear of losing their economic advantage drove the southern states to leave the Union beginning in 1860. The southern states did not want to be controlled by federal laws that threatened their access to the free labor. They also wanted the freedom to travel with their enslaved property without fear of state laws in the North emancipating (freeing) them. When South Carolina's legislature voted to become the first state to secede, or withdraw, from the Union in 1860, it wrote that Lincoln and his Republican Party were "hostile to slavery" and that the "slaveholding states will no longer have the power of self-government, or self-protection, and the Federal Government will have become their enemy." The document listed several other grievances against the federal government, all related to slavery:

> They have denounced as sinful the institution of slavery. They have permitted open establishment among them of societies [referring to abolitionist organizations] whose avowed object is to disturb the peace and to erode the property of the citizens of other states.
>
> They have encouraged and assisted thousands of our slaves to leave their homes and those who remain, have been incited by emissaries,[1] books and pictures to servile insurrection.

To the southern states, it seemed slavery was doomed. Most of the northern states had banned it by the early 1800s. They believed it was only a matter of time before the federal government would make the institution illegal in the South. One by one, the remaining southern states followed South Carolina's lead and seceded from the Union. In their secession documents, each cited the right to preserve the institution of slavery as the motivation behind their decision to leave. Together, these states became known as the Confederacy.

Once the Civil War began, enslaved people resisted their forced labor in even larger numbers. Often, when the Union Army arrived in a Confederate city, enslaved people would run away or join up with the army. When the Union Army occupied New Iberia

---

1. Agents of the federal government sent to represent the government's position or interest.

in April 1861, thousands of enslaved people simply walked away from the plantations, small farms, and town businesses that had kept them in bondage. For them, the war meant freedom at last. They viewed President Lincoln and the Union Army as heroes. Later, when Union forces left New Iberia, bound for New Orleans and Port Hudson, thousands of enslaved people left with them. They traveled on foot and by wagon, horse, and mule. By some accounts, the wagon train was almost ten miles long, made up of more than six thousand soldiers, self-emancipated Africans, and White citizens. Most of the Whites in the caravan were poor and non-slaveholders, fleeing the destruction of war. Although all were refugees, only the Whites were labeled as such. The formerly enslaved people were considered captured Confederate property.

The official end of the Civil War came when General Robert E. Lee surrendered the Confederate Army to Union General Ulysses S. Grant at the Appomattox Courthouse in Virginia on April 9, 1865. The war's end had immediate impacts on enslaved Africans. First, it led to the freeing of millions of formerly enslaved people. Second, it triggered a massive search among the newly freed people for loved ones who had been separated from them during enslavement. Finally, it launched a mass migration of freedmen away from the South.

Reconstructing the South

Following the end of the Civil War, many planters and former slaveholders found themselves penniless once there was no one to work the plantations for free. They could no longer raise the sugarcane crops that once provided them with their great wealth. Moreover, many of their fields and crops had been destroyed in the fighting. In contrast, the human beings enslaved on southern plantations found themselves with few, if any, personal belongings and no money. Even though their labor had created huge wealth for White families, they themselves had nothing. So, the federal government began the task of rebuilding the South and providing additional aid for its people. This period is known as Reconstruction.

In 1865 the federal government created the Bureau of Freedmen, Refugees, and Abandoned Lands. The Freedmen's Bureau, as it came to be called, provided aid to all refugees, regardless of race, who needed food, shelter, fuel, and clothing. (During Reconstruction, the government referred to all Black people as "freedmen," regardless of gender or status prior to the war.)

In many ways Reconstruction was a time of great progress for formerly enslaved people, but also a time of great danger. Many had nowhere to go once they left their former plantations. At the end of the war, freedmen and Whites alike were forced to forage for food and other supplies to avoid starvation. Formerly enslaved people also faced violence from southerners who were angry about losing the war and their way of life. Two years after the creation of the Freedmen's Bureau, Congress passed the Reconstruction Act of March 1867. This legislation allowed the federal government to send troops to oversee the rebuilding of the South's economy. The soldiers would also protect the millions of formerly enslaved men, women, and children of the South.

In the years after the war, many northerners traveled to southern states to take advantage of the ruined southern economies. Most former plantation owners could not manage their farms alone, and many were forced to sell their estates to pay taxes and other debts. Seeing an opportunity to get good land for cheap, these speculators bought up southern land and businesses. The former Confederates deeply disliked these outsiders and referred to them as "carpetbaggers" due to the type of bags they used to travel to the South. During Reconstruction, the term was derogatory, meant to be insulting.

Carpetbaggers were also hated in the South because they typically belonged to the Republican Party. Often called "the party of Lincoln," the nineteenth-century Republican Party wanted citizenship for the freedmen. Citizenship included the right to vote and hold office. By contrast, former Confederates and slaveholders made up much of the nineteenth-century Democratic Party. The Democrats wanted to return the freedmen to the state of slavery, or as close as they could get to it. However, because the federal government was in charge of Reconstruction, the Republican Party controlled the South, at least for a time.

Another derogatory term popular among southerners during Reconstruction was "scalawag." Scalawags were White southerners who remained loyal to the Union during the war. They generally supported the Republican Party and Reconstruction.

Amending the Constitution

Reconstruction was a dangerous time in US history, filled with political fighting and racial hatred. However, it was also a time of great advancement for the freedmen. Shortly after the war ended, Congress began working on changing the national laws to guarantee of freedom, citizenship, and male suffrage (the right to vote). In the end, they passed three amendments to the Constitution, which came to be called the Reconstruction Amendments.

Congress officially ended slavery in 1865 with the passage of the Thirteenth Amendment to the Constitution. Ratified (or passed) on December 6, 1865, the amendment freed all enslaved people in the United States and its territories:

> Neither slavery nor involuntary servitude, except as a punishment for crime whereof the party shall have been duly convicted, shall exist within the United States, or any place subject to their jurisdiction.

Next, Congress ratified the Fourteenth Amendment on July 9, 1868. This granted citizenship to all persons either born in the United States or naturalized (granted citizenship):

> All persons born or naturalized in the United States subject to the jurisdiction thereof, are citizens of the United States wherein they reside. No State shall make or enforce any law which shall abridge the privileges or immunities of citizens of the United States; nor shall any State deprive any person of life, liberty, or property, without due process of law; nor deny to any person within its jurisdiction the equal protection of the laws.

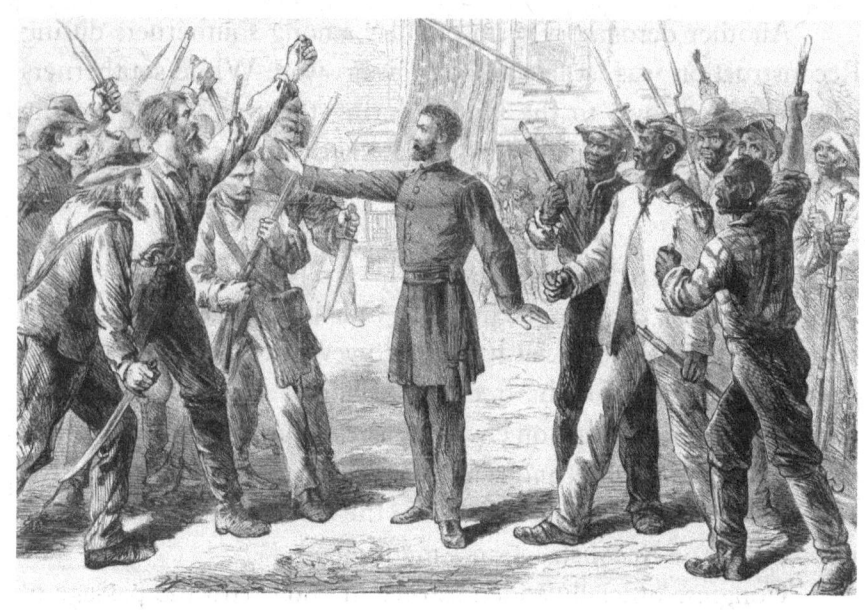

The Freedmen's Bureau by A. R. Waud, 1868.

Source: Library of Congress.

This meant that when she was born in 1868, Emma became the first Wakefield to be born a citizen of the United States.

Following that, the Fifteenth Amendment, ratified February 3, 1870, guaranteed all men the right to vote:

> The right of citizens of the United States to vote shall not be denied or abridged by the United States or by any State on account of race, color, or previous condition of servitude.

Unfortunately, the Fifteenth Amendment did not ban discrimination based on gender. Only male citizens of the United States (regardless of race) were guaranteed suffrage. So, Emma, her mother, and sisters could not vote. However, her father and brothers (once they reached legal age) were guaranteed that right under this amendment. Women around the country would not be granted the right to vote until the Nineteenth Amendment was ratified in 1920.

Thanks to these amendments, the Reconstruction period saw the election of Black men to Congress and to local and state offices. The most prominent in Louisiana were P. B. S. Pinchback, the state's first Black governor, and Oscar Dunn, Louisiana's first Black lieutenant governor. Emma's father, Samuel Wakefield, was elected to public office during this period, first as a member of the mayor's Board of Trustees for the City of New Iberia. Later, he was elected state senator (1874–1876) representing senate district 14, which included Iberia Parish.

Reconstruction Ends

Unfortunately, this period of freedom and relative equality for Black people would not last. Facing pressure from southern representatives, Congress ended the Freedmen's Bureau in 1872. Then, in 1877, Rutherford B. Hayes became president. Although he was a Republican, he had nearly lost to Democrat Samuel Tilden. So, as a compromise, Hayes ordered the federal army to leave the South. This meant that there would be no more protection for Black Americans in the southern states. Reconstruction was over.

Almost immediately, these states began to pass laws that restricted or limited the rights and freedoms of African American citizens. All people of African ancestry were impacted. White southerners began passing laws, codes, and ordinances that segregated, or separated, its citizens based on race. Police officers, sheriffs, and armed White mobs were used to enforce segregation and to "keep Negroes in their place." (The term *Negro* is today considered offensive, though it was commonly used at the time.) These enforcers used threats, false imprisonment, beatings, torture, and lynchings to maintain the social order. A lynching is when a mob puts someone to death, often by hanging, without legal authority to do so.

By 1890, this period of legal and violent segregation came to be known as the Jim Crow Era. The name Jim Crow came from a song in a nineteenth-century minstrel show. Minstrel shows were a form of racist entertainment popular in the nineteenth and early twentieth century. These shows depicted African Americans in skits, songs, and dances using White performers whose faces were usually painted black. The minstrel shows always exaggerated the speech, dress, behavior, and work ethic of Blacks, making fun of them for laughs.

Freedmen were left at the mercy of southern racists and their allies, who successfully preserved segregation for one hundred more years. They intentionally violated the constitutional rights of African American citizens and passed numerous laws to keep Black people from voting. The Jim Crow Era saw the rise of White supremacist groups like the Ku Klux Klan. The Klan used violence, such as lynchings, torture, and cross-burnings, to scare and control African Americans. These actions were part of a system designed to promote White supremacy, keep Black people from making progress, and maintain racism in everyday life.

It is in this time of fear and unfair treatment that Emma Wakefield grew up and earned her medical degree. Even though she faced many challenges and discrimination, she worked hard and succeeded far beyond what anyone expected.

Poetic Forms and Inspirations

Anaphora: The repetition of a word or phrase for an emotional effect. It is often used in poems and speeches, most famously in Dr. Martin Luther King, Jr.'s "I Have a Dream" speech. See "We, the People," page 13, and "I Know Who I Am," page 89.

Ballad: A traditional folktale song usually narrating a tragic story. The form is written in quatrains (stanzas of four lines) with an alternating rhyme scheme (abab). See "Ballad for Sammie," page 35.

Duplex: A form created by Pulitzer Prize-winning poet Jericho Brown. The form combines jazz and sonnet in a seven-couplet, repetitive verse. The first line is echoed in the last line. "Making a Choice" on page 41 is a duplex poem.

Eintou: An African American septet, or a poem of seven lines. *Eintou* is a West African word meaning pearl, as in "pearls of wisdom." The form has a syllable count of 2, 4, 6, 8, 6, 4, 2. See "Wedding Eintou," page 63.

Free Verse: A form of poetry that can be narrative, without a rhyme scheme and meter. Free verse poems do utilize poetic elements but can freely flow without attention to a syllable count or other restrictions of set poem forms. For example, "San Francisco, 1901," "Some People Say," and "Riding Home on the Streetcar."

Golden Shovel: First inspired by Terrance Hayes in a poem he wrote to honor Gwendolyn Brooks. Nikki Grimes further investigates this form in her book *One Last Word*.[1] "The idea of the Golden Shovel poem," writes Grimes, "is to take a short poem in its entirety, or a line from that poem (called a striking line), and

---

1. Nikki Grimes, *One Last Word: Wisdom From the Harlem Renaissance* (London: Bloomsbury, 2017).

create a new poem, using the words from the original. Say you decide to use a single line: you would arrange that line, word by word, in the right margin." The next step is writing "a new poem, each line ending in one of these words." "Aurora Hail, and All the Thousand Dies" (page 27) is a golden shovel using a line from Phillis Wheatley's poem "An Hymn to the Morning," published in 1773.

An Hymn to the Morning
Phillis Wheatley

ATTEND my lays, ye ever honour'd nine,
Assist my labours, and my strains refine;
In smoothest numbers pour the notes along,
For bright Aurora now demands my song.
Aurora hail, and all the thousand dies,
Which deck thy progress through the vaulted skies:
The morn awakes, and wide extends her rays,
On ev'ry leaf the gentle zephyr plays;
Harmonious lays the feather'd race resume,
Dart the bright eye, and shake the painted plume.
Ye shady groves, your verdant gloom display
To shield your poet from the burning day:
Calliope awake the sacred lyre,
While thy fair sisters fan the pleasing fire:
The bow'rs, the gales, the variegated skies
In all their pleasures in my bosom rise.
See in the east th' illustrious king of day!
His rising radiance drives the shades away—
But Oh! I feel his fervid beams too strong,
And scarce begun, concludes th' abortive song.

Source: Phillis Wheatley, *Poems on Various Subjects, Religious and Moral* (London: A. Bell, 1773).

"With tears and toiling breath, for Amelia" (page 31) is another golden shovel using a line from a poem written by Ronald Ross in August 1897. He wrote the poem after he discovered malaria parasites in *anopheline* mosquitoes. Sir Ross received the Nobel Prize in 1902 for his discovery.

> This day relenting God
> Hath placed within my hand
> A wondrous thing; and God
> Be praised. At His command,
> Seeking His secret deeds
> With tears and toiling breath,
> I find thy cunning seeds,
> O million-murdering Death.
> I know this little thing
> A myriad men will save.
> O Death, where is thy sting?
> Thy victory, O Grave?

Source: Ronald Ross, "7. Reply," *In Exile,* section 6, (London: Harrison & Sons, 1931), 73.

Praise Poem: A way to celebrate and honor a person in a poem. "Today I Will Praise," page 84, is a praise poem.

Question Poem: Verse written as questions that are usually unanswerable. "Riding the Train in the Dark" on page 61 is an example of a question poem.

Sestina: Sestina comes from the Latin word for six. It is a complex form that repeats six end words in a specific order in six stanzas with an ending *envoi,* three lines that use all six words. The rules of the form follow a strict repetition pattern. "Graduation Sestina," page 55, is an example of this form.

Thirteen Ways: Originating from "Thirteen Ways of Looking at a Blackbird" by Wallace Stevens, published in 1917. Described as "sensations," the thirteen ways form collects small individual poems that change the reader's perspective with each verse. "Thirteen Ways of Looking at Cholera," page 77, borrows this form.

Sonnet: A classical poetry form that dates back to the thirteenth century. William Shakespeare popularized the form. There are three quatrains (stanzas of four lines each) with a concluding couplet (two lines). The end words of every other line rhyme, except in the final couplet, the two lines rhyme. See "Sonnet after the San Francisco Earthquake, 1906" on page 83.

Ode: A lyrical form that often addresses and celebrates a person, place, thing, or idea. Pablo Neruda popularized the ode with multiple poems about ordinary objects. The ode leads to a revelation about the object of the ode. "Ode to the Steam Locomotive: 1900," page 62, is an example.

Educational Guide

contributed by Linda Mitchell

"The most important thing we can do as teachers, librarians, and human beings is to bear witness."
—author Steven Watkins

"Were You There" is a spiritual sung before its lyrics and music were published in 1899. The repeated question, "Were you there? Were you there? Were you there?" during the tortuous death of Christ prompts singers and audience alike to imagine themselves as witnesses to the Biblical crucifixion.

Were You There? A Biography of Emma Wakefield-Paillet also prompts readers' knowledge and imagination of long-ago Louisiana. Many readers, even those from Dr. Paillet's birthplace of New Iberia, have never heard a thing about her. But if readers could have been there, in the life and times of Dr. Paillet, what would they see? What would they do, based on what they could see? Would readers see strength and resilience, determination to succeed through education? Would they have comforted Dr. Paillet in her many personal losses? Would they have helped her or her family survive and thrive as they changed from enslavement to educated citizens, leaders, and members of society in a Post-Reconstruction and Jim Crow Louisiana? What would any of us do then—and what do we do now?

This nonfiction historical work of Phebe Hayes and Margaret Simon offers readers a carefully researched biography in conversation with poems about the life and legacy of Dr. Emma Wakefield-Paillet, Louisiana's first trained and working female physician. As you read, find out what it was like for young Emma to grow up at such a difficult time in American history. Celebrate her auspicious birth, follow her as she grows and studies, accomplishes and breaks barriers.

Additional Educational Resources

Louisiana History:
Amistad Research Center
The Creole Genealogical and Historical Association
The Historic New Orleans Collection
The Iberia African American Historical Society
Louisiana Endowment for the Humanities and *64 Parishes*
The Whitney Plantation

National History:
The 1619 Project
Black Education, History, and Heritage Alliance at blackpast.org
National Museum of African American History and Culture

Poetry:
Academy of American Poets: Teach this Poem

    Linda Mitchell is a middle school teacher-librarian in Prince William County, Virginia. She holds a master's in social studies education from the State University of New York at Geneseo and a certificate in school library from the University of Virginia College at Wise. She enjoys her family, traveling to historical sites, reading, and creative writing.

Critical Thinking Questions by Section

Meets Common Core State Standards:

- CCSS.ELA-LITERACY.RH.6–8.4. Determine the meaning of words and phrases as they are used in a text, including vocabulary specific to domains related to history/social studies.

- CCSS.ELA-LITERACY.RH.6–8.7. Integrate visual information (e.g., in charts, graphs, photographs, videos, or maps) with other information in print and digital texts.

- CCSS.ELA-LITERACY.RH.6–8.9. Analyze the relationship between a primary and secondary source on the same topic.

- CCSS.ELA-LITERACY.WHST.6–8.10. Write routinely over extended time frames (time for reflection and revision) and shorter time frames (a single sitting or a day or two) for a range of discipline-specific tasks, purposes, and audiences.

Instructions:
As you read through the book, answer the questions below on a separate sheet of paper.

Preface
1. The authors state in the preface, "While prose can tell a story, poetry can touch an emotion." From that sentence, what do you think the authors' purpose is? What do you expect to learn and feel in this story?

2. Have you ever passed by a state historical marker sign and stopped to see what information it offers? History is all around us. The people, places, and ideas of the past can speak to us through those information markers. Find a marker in your area and go read it or look up historical

markers on your state government's website. Find a piece of history close to you. Respond to your experience in writing.

3. Conduct an internet search for the original lyrics of "Were You There." Why do you think the authors chose to echo these lyrics in the title and first poem of the book? What do you learn about Emma Wakefield-Paillet right away from that poem?

The Birth of Emma Wakefield
1. What was new the year you were born? What other person, place or idea has grown up with you?

An Industrious Father
1. What does it mean to be industrious? Describe a time you or someone in your family has shown industriousness.

2. The poem "Under the Swaying Sugarcane" offers this line: "Every day he climbs another rung of the ladder / My father tastes success." What are the rungs on the ladder of success for you? For your family?

The Importance of Education
1. If you built a school, what classes would you offer? Make a list of five to ten classes students in your school could enroll in.

2. Review the list of classes you created. Share with a partner. Do you and your partner have similar or different classes? Combine your lists to create a class catalog for a school. Once a student graduates from the school you and your friend create, what will they be prepared to do as a graduate?

A Family Familiar with Death
1. When someone we know dies, it's customary to send a card or note of sympathy. Create a sympathy card for Emma and her family after the death of one of their family members. Your card should specify who died, words of sympathy, as well as an offer of help you would be prepared to make for Emma during the difficult time after their loved one's death.

2. The authors make clear that Emma was able to recover from the deaths of her father and brother. What do you think helped Emma recover? When you have difficult times, who helps you recover? Write a short note of thanks to this person in your life.

Malaria Claims Sister Amelia
1. Emma's sister Amelia contracted a fatal disease. What diseases exist today that researchers are looking for ways to cure and eradicate?

2. The poem "With tears and toiling breath, for Amelia" is a golden shovel. A golden shovel begins with a "striking line" taken from someone else's work. Find a line or quote from someone else's work you would use in a golden shovel poem.

Another Tragedy Strikes
1. President Biden signed the Emmett Till Anti-Lynching Bill into law on March 29, 2022. Conduct an internet search of the president's comments given at the signing ceremony. Read the transcript or watch the video. Who was Emmett Till, and why is the anti-lynching bill named after him? Name other Civil Rights leaders mentioned in the president's remarks and others at the bill signing ceremony.

2. Violence is part of our world today. What individuals and groups do you know of that are working to reduce and end violence? Write an editorial article expressing your opinion about problems of violence and your ideas about social justice.

3. Saying goodbye is sometimes difficult, sometimes refreshing. The last three lines of "They Come for Adolph" are: "We're packing it in / boarding the train / leaving this place of sin." Have you ever had to say goodbye to a place? Have you ever had to say goodbye to a group of people (maybe your classmates at the end of last school year)? What did it feel like to move on? Were you happy or sad about it?

Embracing Education
1. The ideas we embrace as children and teens become part of our adult experience. What are you embracing today that you hope will be an important part of your future life?

2. Sometimes, choices have to be made when deciding on a career path. Emma had two areas of expertise that she could have chosen. She decided on medicine but as the poem "Making a Choice" suggests in the last lines, "I have a song that plays inside my head." What song from your life holds a message or melody that you will hold onto?

Emma Becomes a Physician
1. "Emma entered medical school at the right time." Sometimes career opportunities open up at just the right time. What career are you thinking about for your future? Is this a career with a long history? Or is this a career that is new due to a need in society? Describe how a career choice that you are thinking of serves our society today. How is this occupation helpful to others?

2. Emma was a first in her state of Louisiana. What would you like to be first to do? Write a few sentences about that. Consider what you would need to learn to be the first.

The Wakefields Leave Louisiana

1. When the Wakefields leave Louisiana, Emma seems to have either been assigned or chosen a new identity in California. If you could go to a new place where nobody knew you or anything about you, where would you go? What aspects of your identity would you keep? What new aspects of identity would you take on?

2. A poem in this section, "Ode to the Steam Locomotive: 1900," celebrates this mode of transportation. Which mode of transportation are you thankful for? Celebrate it with a few lines of praise . . . an ode!

Another Sister Lost

1. In 1902, there were few treatments for conditions such as epilepsy as there are today. Conduct an internet search of advances in medicine since 1900. Describe a condition that once was fatal but is now either cured or survivable with medical help.

Cholera Claims Adolph Wakefield

1. Emma's brother, Adolph, enters the army and "rises through the ranks." Do you think Adolph saw the military as a "ladder of success?" Why do you think yes or no? Discuss with a classmate.

2. The military, especially during wartime like the Spanish-American War, is a dangerous career. Families that see loved ones join the military send notes of love and support during an enlistment. Imagine being Emma in 1899. Write a short note of sisterly love and support to Adolph using details from the time period described in the book.

Returning to Louisiana
1. The poem, "Today I will Praise" is an emotional tribute to Emma's mother. Read the poem carefully and slowly. Notice the line, "Praise the gift of my name." Have you ever considered your name as a gift? Explain how your name is a gift that you appreciate or would like to exchange for another.

2. The death of her mother must have had a significant impact on Emma. Additionally, there was a major earthquake where Emma was living in 1906. It's not clear why Emma returned to New Orleans in 1906 to practice medicine. After such a tumultuous time in her life, imagine what advice Emma might give to new doctors in 1908 about how to be a good doctor.

The End of Emma's Life
1. Now that you have read the book, *Were You There? A Biography of Emma Wakefield-Paillet*, what does the phrase "bearing witness" mean to you? Do you feel that you have borne witness to the life of Emma Wakefield-Paillet? What do you want those who've never heard of her to know?

Pre-Reading and Post-Reading Word Sort

Meets Common Core State Standards:

- CCSS.ELA-LITERACY.RH.6–8.4. Determine the meaning of words and phrases as they are used in a text, including vocabulary specific to domains related to history/social studies.

- CCSS.ELA-LITERACY.RH.6–8.10. By the end of grade 8, read and comprehend history/social studies texts in the grades 6–8 text complexity band independently and proficiently.

- CCSS.ELA-LITERACY.RH.6–8.7. Integrate visual information (e.g., in charts, graphs, photographs, videos, or maps) with other information in print and digital texts.

Instructions:
Before reading *Were You There*, sort the lists of people, places, institutions, and ideas into two groups: "Terms I Know" and "Terms I Don't Know." As you read, move terms you learn from the "Don't Know" column to the "Know" column. When you finish the book, use the book's Historical Background and Poetic Forms and Inspirations to learn about any words that you do not yet know.

People

Frederick Douglass	Phillis Wheatley	William McKinley
We the People	Ronald Ross	Oscar Dunn
Coroner	Dr. James McCune Smith	Abraham Lincoln
Senator	Dr. Rebecca Lee Crumpler	

Names and People I Know	Names and People I Don't Know

117

Places

New Orleans
Avery Island
The Basin Canal

Cuba
San Francisco
Port Hudson

I Know What and Where These Places Are	Places I Don't Know

Institutions / Ideas / Things

Straight University
Reconstruction
Jim Crow Era
Freedman's Bureau
Malaria
Cholera

Music conservatory
Census
Spanish-American War
Epilepsy
Thirteenth Amendment
Antebellum Period

Abolition
Manumission
Suffrage
Fourteenth Amendment
Fifteenth Amendment

Institutions/Ideas/Things I Know	Institutions/Ideas/Things I Don't Know

Going Further:

Without spoilers, discuss your review of the book with someone who is considering reading it.

Timeline Activity

Meets Common Core State Standards:

- CCSS.ELA-LITERACY.W.7.10. Write routinely over extended time frames (time for research, reflection, and revision) and shorter time frames (a single sitting or a day or two) for a range of discipline-specific tasks, purposes, and audiences.

Instructions:

Historians provide timelines as tools to help readers understand a span of time. In *Were You There?* a timeline of Emma's life records major events in her life from her birth to death. Create a timeline of your life inspired by these chapter titles from your birth to today.

Were You There?
Your Life

_____: the birth of _____ (your name)

Parents, Guardians _____

Education _____

A Family Familiar with _____
(My family is familiar with...)

I Know Who I Am :
Something important in your life today.

Synthesis Questions:
1. List several people who bear witness to your life and why they are important witnesses to you.

2. What document, photo, or artifact would you want to help tell your story 150 years from today?

Write a Poem

Meets Common Core State Standards:

- CCSS.ELA-LITERACY.W.6.10. Write routinely over extended time frames (time for research, reflection, and revision) and shorter time frames (a single sitting or a day or two) for a range of discipline-specific tasks, purposes, and audiences.

Instructions:

Many forms of poetry are used in *Were You There*, including:
- Anaphora
- Ballad
- Duplex
- Eintou
- Free Verse
- Golden Shovel
- Praise Poem
- Sestina
- Thirteen Ways
- Sonnet
- Ode

Some poems are written in a specific form and some are in free verse. Some poems are based on words and lyrics from the time Dr. Paillet lived and some contain a more recent connection. Choose one of the poetry forms listed and write a poem that fits the form. Use "Wedding Eintou" from the book as a mentor text. Be sure to include a pearl of wisdom for your readers.

Acknowledgments

I am deeply and forever grateful for the tremendous support of my family and friends as I researched and penned Dr. Wakefield-Paillet's incredible story. I could not have a better husband than Harold Hayes, my loving and supportive spouse of forty-five years. He is the silent partner in all I do for the Iberia African American Historical Society.

I first learned of Dr. Emma Wakefield-Paillet from a story New Orleans historian and genealogist, Jari Honora, posted in his online blog, CreoleGen. Prior to that post, I had never heard of Emma. If it were not for Jari identifying Emma as a New Iberia native who was the first Black woman to graduate with a medical degree in Louisiana, this book would not exist.

A very big "Thank you!" to Kristin Amundsen for sending me pictures of Emma, Joseph, and other family members. Kristin is Joseph Oscar Paillet's several times great-niece.

The staff at the Historic New Orleans Collection, the Dillard University archives, and the Amistad Center were very helpful in the early phase of my research. The board of directors and general members of the Iberia African American Historical Society, of course, were central to the success of this literary project.

By happenstance, I met Emily Robertson Wright and was immediately struck by her son's art. Incarcerated, he expresses his creativity through painting. I thank Clifford Etienne for the cover art.

–Phebe A. Hayes

I am grateful that Phebe Hayes asked me to have coffee with her in 2018 and told me the story of Emma. She entrusted me with the charge to write poetry about Emma's life.

I acknowledge my writing group friend, middle school librarian Linda Mitchell, for donating her time and expertise to create an educational guide.

Thanks to UL Press editor Devon Lord for believing in this work and easing us with her encouraging comments.

I am grateful for my faithful writing group which meets twice a month on Zoom (even before the pandemic): Molly Hogan, Catherine Flynn, Linda Mitchell, Heidi Mordhorst, and Mary Lee Hahn, who read and fell in love with Emma and her story and supported my journey through poetic history.

And always my husband, Jeff, who is my hero every day.

–Margaret G. Simon

About the Authors

PHEBE A. HAYES is a descendant of African families formerly enslaved on nineteenth-century local plantations. Several of her male ancestors were veterans of the Union Army and Navy. She is passionate about humanizing her people by providing evidence of their experiences and contributions to Iberia Parish and surrounding communities, from slavery to the end of Jim Crow segregation.

Phebe is a professor (Department of Communicative Disorders) and dean emerita (College of General Studies) at the University of Louisiana at Lafayette after twenty-seven years of service. After retirement, she founded he Iberia African American Historical Society (IAAHS), located in New Iberia, Louisiana. Through IAAHS, she also organized the Iberia African American Historical Society Center for Research & Learning, an archive of primary documents, civil records, and pictures related to the true and inclusive history of the community.

MARGARET SIMON lives on the Bayou Teche in New Iberia, Louisiana. Margaret has been an elementary school teacher for thirty-six years. She's the author of *Bayou Song: Creative Explorations of the South Louisiana Landscape*. Margaret has contributed to children's anthologies including *The Poetry of US* by National Geographic and *Rhyme & Rhythm: Poems for Student Athletes*. Margaret writes a blog regularly at http://reflectionsontheteche.com.